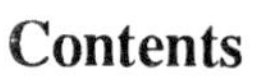

Contents

Current Approaches

Advances in Pancreatitis

Edited by
P L Zentler-Munro & V J Harten Ash

duphar
medical relations

First published 1989

ISBN 1-870678-13-3

Printed and bound in Great Britain by
Inprint (Litho) Ltd., Southampton
Tel 0703 227435.

EDITOR'S FOREWARD

Acute pancreatitis is still a significant cause of death in young people, and chronic pancreatitis ofter causes terrible suffering and disability. Our understanding of the physiology of the pancreas, gathered largely from animal studies, is advancing rapidly. Our knowledge of the pathophysiology of pancreatic disease lags far behind, partly because it can be gained only by the study of a relatively inaccessible organ in a notoriously heterogeneous group of patients. Our knowledge of the treatment of pancreatic disease is primitive indeed - either we have no hypotheses to test, or we do not know how to test them.

In Autumn 1988 a group of physicians and surgeons with special interests in inflammatory diseases of the pancreas met to discuss these problems at the Royal College of Physicians. A working knowledge of the area was assumed, and each speaker was asked to present those aspects of his subject which seemed most to merit attention now. This publication contains these "state of the art" presentations, together with the lively and constructive discussion that followed, edited to achieve unity of format and to avoid overlap.

The first part of the book considers acute pancreatitis. Dr Keynes discusses the controversial role of bacterial infection in primary pathogenesis, as yet little exploited in therepeutic research. Mr Imrie then assesses recent developments in the clinical and laboratory identification of the patient most at risk from an acute attack, and Dr Chalmers presents a promising new method using dynamic CT scanning. This leads the way for Dr Salmon to review the confusing array of medical treatments on offer - here, more than anywhere else, we are still limited by the lack of adequate controlled clinical trials. The surgeons have been more productive in this area, and Mr. Neoptolemos contributes a comprehensive review of the somewhat sounder basis for endoscopic surgery in gallstone pancreatitis.

The second part of the book considers chronic pancreatitis. Mr McMahon analysis the various mechanisms by which alcohol may damage the pancreas - a well-established effect which is still surprisingly poorly understood. Dr Boyd reviews the current role of pancreatic function tests in chronic pancreatitis, which have perhaps still to meet the demands we would like to make of them. Mr Russell presents a sanguine overview of the widely differing practice of surgery in chronic pancreatitis, and Dr Zentler-Munro ends by proposing a physiological model of medical therapy requiring exploitation in clinical trials and practice.

We hope this book offers a succinct and entertaining summary of the growing points in pancreatic inflammatory disease. We would like to thank Duphar Ltd for their enterprise in organising the meeting, and their generous sponsorship of this book

Patrick L Zentler-Munro
Consultant Physician
Raigmore Hospital
Inverness

BACTERIOLOGY AND ACUTE HAEMORRHAGIC PANCREATITIS

Mr Milo Keynes
Cambridge

In the first description of acute haemorrhagic pancreatitis (HP) in 1889, Fitz argued that the disease was caused by a bacterial infection spreading from the duodenum by reflux along the pancreatic duct.(1) Opie disagreed (2) (3) (4); based on two patients of his own and the reports on five others in the literature, Opie considered that because of the variable and inconstant results of bacterial culture, the various organisms found in the necrotic pancreatic tissue were not aetiological agents, but merely opportunistic invaders of injured tissue. His other postulates also derived from the same seven patients. Earlier, Flexner had shown that intraductal injection of various organisms caused the 'haemorrhagic inflammation' of acute pancreatitis (AP) (5) but, as a result of Opie's book in 1903, there has been strikingly little research into the possibility that bacterial infection might play a part in the pathogenesis of AP. There has been a lack of bacterial data from preconceived theories that HP is purely due to chemical autodigestion (which it is not), though the aseptic nature of necrotic pancreatitis is far from proven. (6)

Experimentally, it has been shown many times that intraductal injection of bile was more likely to produce pancreatitis if the bile was infected than if it were sterile. (6) Armstrong, Taylor and Torrance injected the pancreatic ducts of rats with sterile bile under low pressure, and with infected bile after passing it through a filter, without producing HP; but injection of bile infected with E.coli produced HP (7). In 1956, it was noticed that not all bacteria can give HP on intraductal injection, but only those that produce toxins that can damage cell-membrane phospholipids and give an intradermal necrotising lesion. (8) The production of experimental HP by bacteria is dependent on organisms that produce cytotoxins, and is preventable by immunisation, antitoxins, or antibiotics. (6) (8).

The Pfeffer closed duodenal loop has been widely used since 1957 for studying AP, but recently it has been called an 'inappropriate model' that should be abandoned because infection as well as AP occurs. (9) (10) This preparation can, however, produce HP even in germ-free dogs.(11) In 87 dogs given blind loops, 67% developed HP, and 10% acute interstitial pancreatitis (IP), but only when reflux occurred. (12) In 4 dogs with IP, both loop fluid and pancreas were sterile, but, in 6 with HP, there were similar high bacterial counts in the loop fluid and in the pancreas. (12) Intraductal injection of infected loop fluid gave HP, but when filtered, gave IP. In the dogs with HP, but not these with IP, there were high levels of plasma amidase, levels that were lowered by treatment with neomycin (but not with intravenous aprotinin). There was a correlation between pancreatic infection, HP and raised levels of the proteolytic amidase. Amidase showed a broad specificity and stability uncharacteristic of pancreatic proteases, but similar to the bacterial enzyme preparation pronase which can cause intradermal necrosis. (12)

AP may follow ERCP, and in some patients the pancreatitis has been associated with infection introduced by the endoscope. (13) Gregg found that bacteria, usually Gram negative, were present in the pancreatic juice of a third of patients with AP, and that in those with infected juice the clinical course was particularly severe. (14) Infected bile may also be a cause of HP, and one report found that 14.4% of patients with biliary pancreatitis also had acute cholangitis and that 23.3% with gallstone-related cholangitis showed AP. (15) These patients developed pancreatitis from reflux of bacteria, despite anti-bacterial activity of pancreatic juice to many 'gut' organisms. (16)

Clinically, the bacteria grown from pancreatic abscesses, or necrotic pancreas, are invariably cytotoxin producers and likely to be Gram negative 'gut' organisms. (6) Beger and his colleagues explored 209 patients with HP, and found microorganisms, usually E. coli, in the necrotic pancreatic tissue in 85, (40.7%). (17) (18) In a group with pancreatic sepsis explored within 21 days of onset, the mortality was 61%, compared with 5.9% in those with sterile necrosis. (17) In another study using percutaneous computed tomography-guided aspiration, 40% of patients with HP had pancreatic infection (19).

No adequate clinical trials have been performed to evaluate the use of antibiotics in AP, but their apparent failure to affect the course of the disease has strengthened the assumption that the infection is a secondary event. Patients with HP have, however, a high mortality rate despite all treatment, whereas those with IP are likely to survive with only supportive therapy; unless the distinction is made in each patient, a trial is unlikely to prove useful.

The clinical courses of HP and those of septic shock, toxic syndrome, Gram negative septicaemia and endotoxaemia show similarities, and experimentally oxygen-derived free radicals and endotoxins may cause HP. In patients with AP, the degree of endotoxaemia correlates with the severity of the attack. (6) (18)

These observations only suggest, and cannot be interpretated as firm evidence of, a primary bacterial role in the developmnet of HP. But, in those with infected pancreatic necrosis, the infection was sufficiently severe for the exploration to be undertaken within a mean duration from the onset of illness of seven days. (17) (18) Gerzof and his co-workers found that infection could be shown in a majority of patients with pancreatic infection within 14 days of the onset of AP. (20) This could argue for a primary infection rather than rapid, contaminating secondary colonisation.

But does secondary infection take place all that commonly, and how does it occur? Of the 50 of 92 percutaneous aspirates in 60 patients with pancreatic inflammatory masses which proved sterile, none subsequently showed infection. (20) And a total of 124 patients found at operation to have a sterile necrosis were most unlikely to show a later, secondary infection, and, as already pointed out, had a far better survival than those with infected necrotic tissue. (17) (18)

After the necrosis of the blood vessels, initially, secondary infection must be only at the periphery of the necrotic pancreatic tissue. It is hardly satisfactory to assume, and blandly state, that it occurs because there is a diathesis of the 'gut' organisms to infect necrotic pancreas in such patients. There is evidence for translocation of intestinal bacteria into experimental intra-abdominal abscesses, though the way this occurs is not known. (21) It is speculated to be either by way of haematogenous or lymphatic channels, by transmural migration through the cellular layers of the intestine to the periphery of the necrotic tissue, or, most strongly, by the liberation of phagocytosed organisms into the extra-intestinal site. (21)

Opie's assumption that bacteria play no part in the pathogenesis of AP has been challenged. It seems possible that in at least 40% of those with HP it is primary infection by bacteria capable of producing cytotoxins that causes the pancreatic necrosis. The bacteriology of severe AP urgently requires further investigation.

References

1. Fitz RH. Acute pancreatitis: a consideration of pancreatic hemorrhage; hemorrhagic suppurative and gangrenous pancreatitis and disseminated fat necrosis. *Boston Med Surg* J 1889; 120: 181-7; 205-7; 229-35.
2. Opie EL. The etiology of acute hemorrhagic pancreatitis. *Johns Hopkins Hosp Bull* 1901; 12: 182-8.
3. Opie EL. *Disease of the Pancreas - its cause and nature*. Philadelphia: JB Lippincott, 1903.
4. Opie EL, Meakins JC. Data concerning the etiology and pathology of hemorrhagic necrosis of the pancreas. *J Exp Med 1909:* 11: 561-78.
5. Flexner S. Experimental pancreatitis. *Johns Hopkins Hosp Reports1901;9: 743-71.*
6. Keynes M. Heretical thoughts on the pathogenesis of acute pancreatitis. *Gut 1988; 29: 1413-23.*
7. Armstrong CP, Taylor TV, Torrance HB . Pressure, volume and the pancreas. *Gut* 1985; 26: 615-24.
8. Thal AP, Tansathithaya P, Egner W. An experimental study of bacterial pancreatitis. *Surg Gynecol Obstet* 1956; 103: 459-68.
9. Pfeffer RB, Stasior O, Hinton JW. The clinical picture of sequential development of acute hemorrhagic pancreatitis in the dog. *Surg Forum* 1957; 8: 248-51.
10. McMahon MJ. Acute pancreatitis. *Current opinion in Gastroenterology* 1987;3: 698-713.
11. Nance FC, Cain JL. Hemorrhagic pancreatitis in germ free dogs. *Surg Forum 1967; 18: 365-7.*
12. Keynes WM. A non-pancreatic source of the proteolytic-enzyme amidase and bacteriology in experimental pancreatitis. *Ann Surg 1*980; 191: 187 -99.
13. Elson CO, Hattori K, Blackstone MO. Polymicrobial sepsis following endoscopic retrograde cholangiopancreatography. *Gastroenterology 1*975; 69: 507-10.
14. Gregg JA. Detection of bacterial infection of the pancreatic ducts in patients with pancreatitis and pancreatic cancer during endoscopic retrograde cholangiopancreatography. *Gastroenterology 1*977; 73: 1005-7.
15. Neoptolemos JP, Carr-Locke DL, Leese T, James D. Acute cholangitis in association with acute pancreatitis: incidence, clinical features and outcome in relation to ERCP and endoscopic sphincterotomy. *BR J Surg* 1987; 74: 1103-6.
16. Rubinstein E, Mark Z, Haspel J, et al. Antibacterial activity of the pancreatic fluid. *Gastroenterology* 1985; 88: 927-32.
17. Beger HG, Bittner R, Block S, Buchler M. Bacterial contamination of pancreatic necrosis. *Gastroenterology* 1986; 91: 433-8.
18. Beger HG, Buchler M, Bittner R, et al. Necrosectomy and postoperative local lavage in necrotizing pancreatitis. *Br J Surg* 1988; 75: 207-12.

19. Gerzof SG, Banks PA, Spechler SJ, et al. Role of guided percutaneous aspiration in early diagnosis of pancreatic sepsis. *Dig Dis Sci 1*984; 29: 950.
20. Gerzof SG, Banks PA, Robbins AH, et al. Early diagnosis of pancreatic infection by computed tomography-guided aspiration. *Gastroenterology* 1987; 93: 1315-20.
21. Wells CL, Rotstein OD, Pruett TL, Simmons RL. Intestinal bacteria translocate into experimental intra-abdominal abscesses. *Arch Surg* 1986; *121: 102-6.*

DETECTION OF THE HIGH RISK PATIENT: DOES IT MATTER?

Mr C W Imrie
Consultant Surgeon
Glasgow Royal Infirmary

Introduction

The identification of this group is important for focussing attention on those most in need of treatment. An objective grading system is unnecessary for the grossly ill but there is a "grey zone" with patients who are difficult to assess (even by experts) and objective grading factors can be useful. These measurements will also allow a comparison of studies to be carried out from centre to centre. Finally they do allow selection of a group of patients who need to be the main source of study for new therapies, since the 75% who have mild disease tend to get better quickly with standard conservative management.

PROGNOSTIC GRADING SYSTEMS

Accurate grading systems to identify severe acute pancreatitis have been somewhat complex. The original Ranson criteria were based on an analysis of over 40 parameters. (1) We in Glasgow followed this by producing eleven and subsequently eight prognostic factors, chosen deliberately to have European equivalents. (2)(3) McMahon then suggested an assessment using peritoneal free fluid, or returned lavage fluid, comprising simply the clinical picture, the discoloration of the fluid, and the presence of bacterial infection. The Amelie Waring project included over 400 patients in Leeds,Bristol and Glasgow, of whom 91 severely ill patients entered the study (5). The analysis was based on peritoneal aspiration, and in only one patient was return lavage fluid studied the basis for grading severity. Most of the patients were graded at high risk on the presence of at least 20 mls of free fluid and discolouration of aspirate; all patients who died were positive for both these factors.

The Leeds system is valuable in studying those with alcoholic pancreatitis but very poor for gallstone pancreatitis. The Glasgow grading system, on the other hand, is equally good for the two major aetiologies; better than the Leeds aspiration method for gallstone pancreatitis, but less good for alcoholic pancreatitics (6).

Prognostic factors used in New York and Glasgow include white count, the degree of hypoxaemia, LDH elevation, urea and calcium. It is possible to derive a system of weighting with emphasis on these, and less importance attached to other factors: albumin, glucose and age.

Many people are unhappy with the multiple grading systems as they involve much work and are not always possible to perform. The ideal prognostic factor would be a single blood measurement, simple to perform, cheap reproducible, and sensitive and specific. Are we asking for the impossible? Single factor analysis showed that an LDH greater than 600 IU/L, or a serum calcium level of less than 2.0 mM/L uncorrected, or an arterial hypoxaemia of less than 7 kPa was each associated with an elevation in the risk of major complications or death, but none sufficed as a single prognostic factor. Fibrinogen levels of greater than 6 gm/L have been suggested as a valuable marker of severity. (7) We did not find this so in a study of 180 patients (8): levels were higher in patients with severe disease than in those with mild disease, but there was no clear cut off value.

McMahon suggested that C-reactive protein could predict the later complications of acute pancreatitis, sepsis or pseudocyst .(9) The function of this acute phase protein in the body is not understood. It is being used to grade Crohn's disease activity and studies in several other diseases are in progress. Buchler et al in a study of only 35 patients, suggested that C-reactive protein levels greater than 120 mg/L were a 95% discriminator of the presence of acute necrotising pancreatitis. (10) In their study it exceeded the accuracy of CT scanning. Additionally alpha 2 macroglobulin levels less than 150 mg per litre showed an 82% discrimination. Patients with oedematous pancreatitis had low levels of C-reactive protein, and those with necrotising pancreatitis had higher levels, with a good seperation. It is important to note that the initial values in this German study were very high, a questionable response for C reactive protein. A study from Helsinki showed similar features, with a good discrimination between patients with more than 3 prognostic factors on the Ranson system and those with less. (11) But again the initially high levels of C-reactive protein must make the deductions questionable.

Our study at Glasgow Royal Infirmary involved over 70 patients. (11)The C-reactive protein response was as anticipated for an acute phase protein: the mild groups had an elevated level (100 mg/L) by the second and third days. Those who died or developed major complications had a much higher and statistically significant elevation, but the value of C-reactive protein as a good marker of necrosis was not substantiated. Patients with major respiratory complications had a pattern similar to the patients who developed necrosis or pseudocyst. Additionally we would suggest that levels of150mg/L or more (rather than 100 mg/L) better identify those patients with the most severe disease. The initial rise in the first 12 hours however restricts its use. From 30 hours onwards the results are very valuable indeed in distinguishing the two groups of patients. C-reactive protein is a cheap, reproducible test and the results are available quickly. It should be employed in conjuction with other objective methods of assessment, such as CT or the Leeds and Glasgow systems, as an early predictor of severe acute pancreatitis but not as an indication of necrotising acute pancreatitis, warranting early surgical intervention. Indeed, in our experience, such use might have harmed patients with respiratory insufficiency, who recovered without surgical intervention.

Assessing Prognosis

There have been suggestions that the use of these systems alone,without clinical assessment might provide an accurate prognosis. No clinician can however shut out the clinical findings. More experienced clinicians are better at discerning the likely prognosis, and such assessments can be good, by 48 hours as good as any of the individual scoring systems which have been used.

The APACHE 2 system (Acute Physiology and Chronic Health Evaluation mark 2) yields a dynamic prognosis picture based on assessment parameters. (12) Originally described about 12 years ago, it has been used extensively in intensive care units over the past 6 years. It can be applied in acute pancreatitis and is particularly valuable from the initial assessment. There is a significant differentiation between the mild cases and the patients who die, again best at 48 hours. Similarly, patients with complications have higher APACHE scores. A score above 8 units tends to indicate a poor prognosis.

Grading in Practice

I use a combination of clinical assessment, the Glasgow prognostic score, the Leeds aspiration method, and C-reactive protein values. Our new CT scanner is yet to be fully installed and so currently is precluded from utilisation in grading the severity of AP.

Future Approaches

Professor Herman-Taylor of St George's Hospital, London, has recently pioneered the measurement of urinary trypsinogen activation peptide(TAP). It is hoped such a measure will relate to the degree of trypsinogen activation and hence to the eventual severity of the acute pancreatitis. From initial work on a group of 60 patients, it appears that there is a good discrimination, being highest in the patients with chronically severe acute pancreatitis, and that there is a better correlation at the initial assessment than with C- reactive protein. It is hoped soon to perform blood assays on the values of TAP with the ultimate hope of a satisfactory rapid test to confirm acute pancreatitis and to provide an accurate index of severity of disease.

References

1. Ranson J H C, Rifkind K M, Roses D F, et al, Prognostic signs and role of operative management in acute pancreatitis. *Surg Gynacol Obstel 1974; 139: 69-81.*
2. Imrie C W, Benjamin I S, Ferguson J C et al. A single centre double blind rialof trasylol therpy in primary acute pancreatitis. *Br J Surg* 1978; 65: 337-341.
3. Osbourne D H, Imrie C W, Carter D C. Biliary surgery at the same admission for gallstone associated pancreatitis. *Br J Surg* 1981; 68: 758-761.
4. Bradley J S, Bradley P, Cameron J L, et al. Diagnostic peritoneal lavage in acute pancreatitis, the value of microscopy of the fluid. *Br J Surg 1981; 68: 245-246.*
5. Mayer A D , McMahon M J, Corfield A P, et al. Controlled clinical trial of peritoneal lavage for the treatment of serere acute pancreatitis. *N Engl J Med* 1985; 372: 399-404.
6. Corfield A P, Cooper M J, Williamson R C N, et al. Prediction of sererity in acute pancreatitis: prospective comparison of three prognostic indices. *Lancet* 1985; ii: 403-7.
7. Berry A R, Taylor T V , Davies E C. Diagnostic tests and prognostic indicators in acute pancreatitis. J *Roy Coll Surg Edinb* 1982; 27; 345-352.
8. Shearer M E, Campbell F C, Walker I D, et al. Plasma fibrinogen levels in acute pancreatitis. *J Roy Coll Surg Edinb* 1985; 30: 245-247.
9. Mayer A D, McMahon M J, Bowen M, et al. C-reactive protein: an aid to assessment and monitoring of acute pancreatitis. J Clin Pathol 1984; 37, 207-11.
10. Buchler M. Malfertheiner P. Beger H G. Correlation of imaging procedures, biochemical parametres and clinical stage in acute pancreatitis. In; Malfertheiner P, Ditschuneit H. eds, Diagnostic procedures in pancreatic disease.Berline: Springer-Verlag, 1986, 123-9.
11. Puolakkainer P, Valtonen V, Paananen A, et al. C-reactive protein (CRP) and serum phospholipase A2 in the assessment of the severity of acute pancreatitis. *Gut* 1987; 28: 764-71.
12. Wilson C. Heads A. Shenkin A, et al. C-reactive protein, antiproteases and complement factors as objective markers of severity in acute pancreatitis. *Br. J. Surg*. 1989; 76: 177-181.
13. Knaus W A. Draper E A, Wagner D P, et al. Apache II: A severity of disease classification system. *Crit Care Med* 1985; 13: 818-829.

PANCREATIC NECROSIS - CAN DYNAMIC COMPUTERISED TOMOGRAPHY HELP IN PATIENT MANAGEMENT?

Dr A G Chalmers
Consultant Radiologist
Leeds General Infirmary

Introduction

The management of patients with severe acute pancreatitis is difficult and at best controversial. In those patients who die, autopsy will demonstrate pancreatic necrosis in the majority. Some authorities argue therefore that the removal of necrotic tissue by debridement offers the only prospect of survival. The decision to operate will be more confidently made if pre-operative imaging can satisfy two basic requirements: the accurate identification of pancreatic necrosis and some indication of its distribution and extent.

The pre-operative diagnosis of pancreatic necrosis proved elusive. It is now accepted that neither clinical assessment, physiological scores, nor diagnostic peritoneal lavage can identify patients with pancreatic necrosis accurately. Ultrasound cannot assess pancreatic viability and CT severity scores, although showing a clear correlation between disease severity and the incidence of pancreatic necrosis, cannot make the specific diagnosis. Even the surgeon at laparotomy often has considerable difficulty in differentiating viable from necrotic tissue.

Dynamic CT

The use of CT in the assessment of acute pancreatitis was at first limited by the reluctance of radiologists and clinicians to use intravenous radiographic contrast media. Non-enhanced scans give similar information to ultrasound - a display of gross pancreatic morphology but no indication of viability. In the last few years, particularly since the development of non-ionic contrast media, work from Scandinavia and Germany has established the role of dynamic contrast-enhanced CT in the pre-operative diagnosis of pancreatic necrosis. The response of the pancreatic parenchyma to contrast, and the patency of adjacent vessels can be clearly seen. Such appearances have led some workers to describe the technique as dynamic angio-CT.

We can attempt to quantify the parenchymal response by using the computer software to calculate the attenuation values within particular regions of interest. The degree of enhancement by contrast can then be assessed by the change in CT number in similar regions before and after contrast. In some centres, particularly in Scandinavia, patients with severe acute pancreatitis are categorised by this response into low and high enhancement groups. Those with 'low enhancement' are considered to have pancreatic necrosis and surgery is recommended, while those with 'high enhancement' are managed conservatively. In other words, clinicians in such centres are placing great emphasis on the CT findings when deciding which of their patients require surgery and which do not. Should we be doing the same?

CT Technique

Oral contrast is given to opacify the small bowel before and between scanning sequences. A pre-contrast non-dynamic series is then performed which documents the extent of extra-pancreatic disease, and identifies the

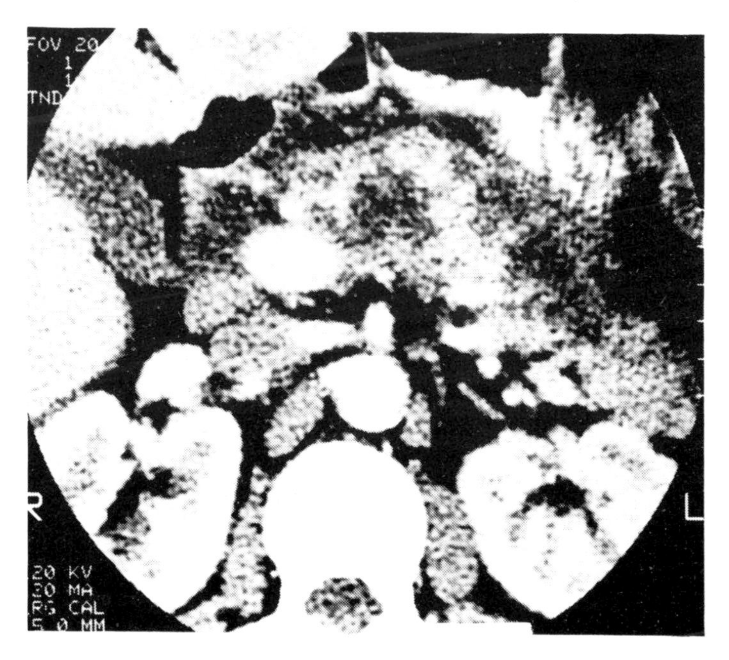

Figure 1: Targetted dynamic post-contrast image through pancreas, in patient with severe acute pancreatitis. Large areas of non-enhancing parenchyma demonstrated between patches of residual viable tissue.

pancreatic levels for the post-contrast dynamic series. Some 10-12 slices are then obtained after the injection of 150mls of non-ionic contrast. In a normal pancreas, there is uniform parenchymal enhancement from head to tail. In oedematous pancreatitis, similar uniform enhancement is generally obtained. In severe necrotising pancreatitis, there are large areas of non- enhancement with only patchy areas of residual viable pancreatic parenchyma (Figure 1).

The value of intravenous contrast is made clear when the pre- and post-contrast images of this patient are viewed together. The pre-contrast image gives no indication of the extent of pancreatic damage displayed following contrast (Figure 2).

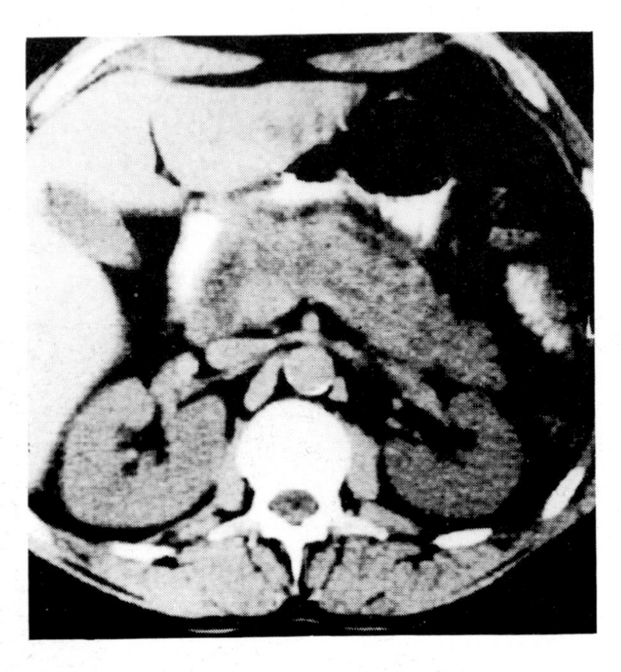

Figure 2: Non-targetted, non-contrast image of pancreas of patient illustrated in Figure 1.

Results of CT Investigation

During the first 18 months of the CT scanner's installation at the General Infirmary at Leeds, Mr McMahon's team prospectively assessed some 32 patients with acute pancreatitis, in whom pancreatic necrosis was suspected. The majority displayed an increase in physiological scores at 5-7days, while the remainder had either overt organ failure or severe disease on ultrasound or CT performed elsewhere. The end points for the study were confirmation of more than 20gms of necrotic pancreas or peripancreatic tissue at laparotomy or autopsy or, when necrosis was not suggested by CT, an uneventful recovery. The decision to operate, it should be stressed, was not based on CT appearance alone but on evidence of clinical deterioration and paticularly sepsis.

Seven cases displayed features consistent with pancreatic necrosis using CT numbers as previously described, and this was confirmed at laparotomy or post mortem in each. Two showed equivocal enhancement which resolved on follow-up scanning and, of the remaining 23, none displayed or subsequently developed evidence of pancreatic necrosis.

In this small series of patients the findings at operation or autopsy confirmed the CT documentation in each case. We therefore agree with other workers that CT can identify pancreatic necrosis accurately and localise its extent precisely.

PATIENT MANAGEMENT

How useful is this information to the clinician managing the patient? Does the CT demonstration of necrosis mean surgery is indicated?

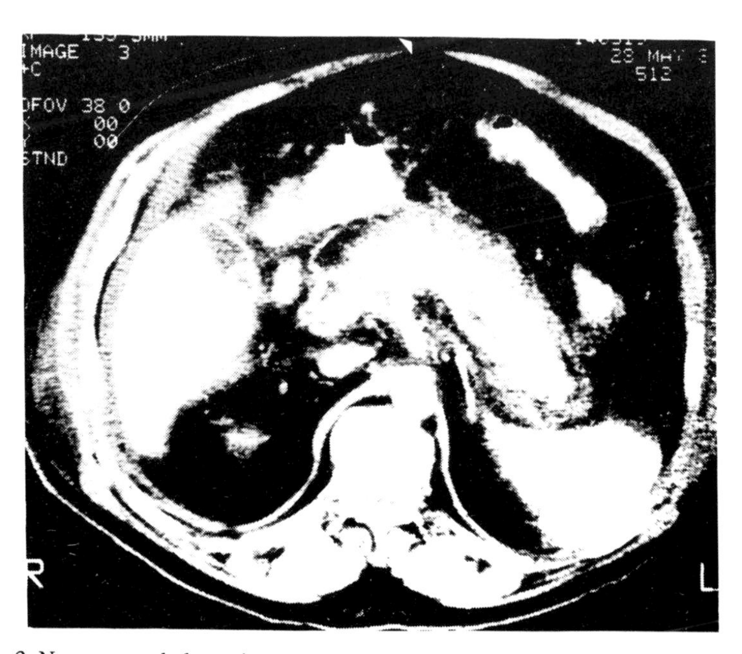

Figure 3: Non-targetted, dynamic post-contrast image in critically ill patient with severe acute pancreatitis. Rim of non-enhancing tissue, anterior to viable parenchyma. Confirmed at subsequent post mortem as peripheral pancreatic parenchymal necrosis.

initial series, and CT demonstrated a rim of tissue anterior to the viable parenchyma, with clearly different attenuation values (Figure 3).

These appearances correlated exactly with those of the pancreas at subsequent post mortem, with a rim of necrotic tissue surrounding the underlying viable pancreas. How one differentiates on CT between peripheral pancreatic parenchymal necrosis and immediate peri-pancreatic fat necrosis I do not know, but I would suggest that such differentiation is unnecesary on clinical grounds.

We have now seen a number of patients with similar CT appearances of predominantly peripheral pancreatic necrosis, who have responded to conservative management and have not required surgical intervention. It appears that the extent of pancreatic necrosis and the associated peripancreatic change as documented by CT do not always correlate with the severity of the illness as assessed clinically. The more cases of acute pancreatitis we scan, the more patients we see who appear very sick radiologically but clinically remain stable and do not require surgery.

A dramatic example of this is illustrated by a 25 year old male with severe acute pancreatitis. The pre-contrast series showed a swollen pancreas with extensive extra-pancreatic disease. The post-contrast films demonstrated large areas of non-enhancing tissue, (Figure 4).

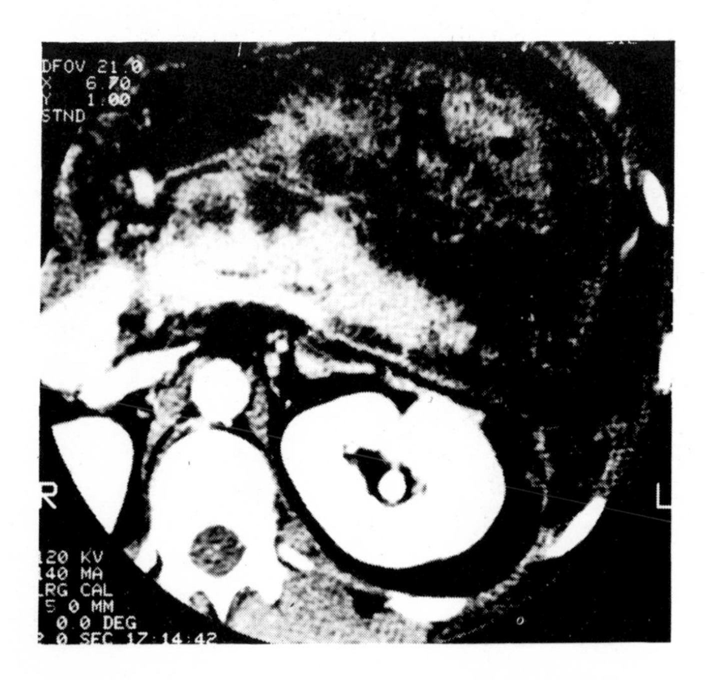

Figure 4: Young man with severe acute pancreatitis. Dynamic post-contrast scan showing residual viable parenchyma, contrasting with large areas of non-enhancement.

The patient responded well to conservative management, surgery was not required. Follow-up scans showed no disease progression and the patient was discharged in due course. The most recent scan at a recent out-patient attendance showed a loss of between a third and a half of his functioning pancreatic parenchyma, but he remains clinically well (Figure 5).

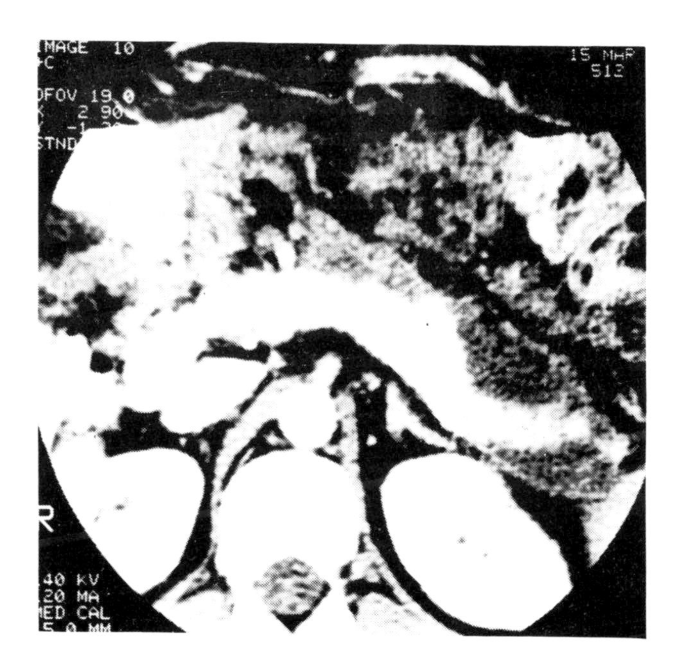

Figure 5: Subsequent out-patient follow-up dynamic scan of patient illustrated in Figure 4. Excellent response to conservative management, clear demonstration of residual viable parenchyma,contrasting with organizing, non-enhancing tissue.

What is the eventual prognosis for patients who display mainly peripheral necrosis? Leaving aside any eventual biochemical deficit,I suspect they may show disturbed pancreatic morphology, with a rim of soft tissue surrounding the pancreas. Biopsies will show changes consistent with previous pancreatic necrosis.

Similar CT appearances can be associated with strikingly different clinical courses illustrated by these two final patients. The first displays extensive pancreatic necrosis with residual islands of viable parenchyma within the head and tail. There were no clinical indications for surgery and this patient is currently walking around a ward in the Infirmary at Leeds in blissful ignorance of these dramatic CT findings (Figure 6a).

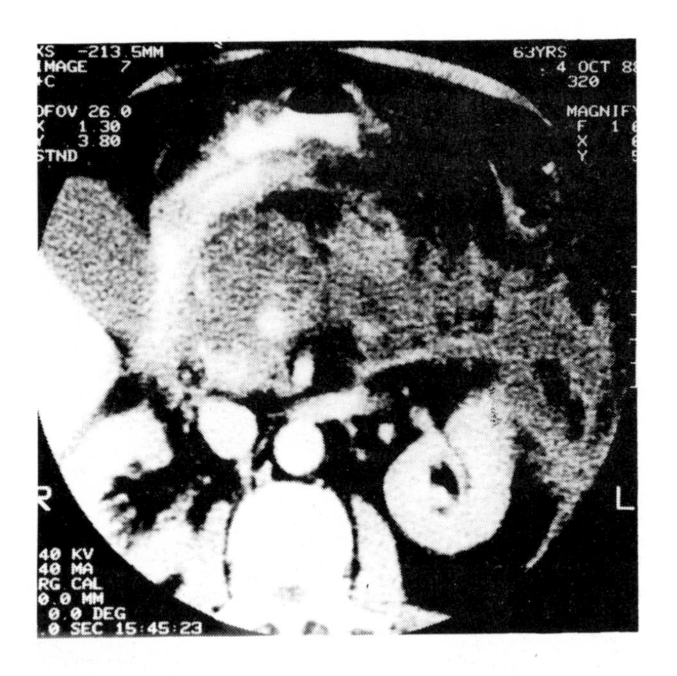

Fig 6a

By way of contrast, a patient with similar CT findings had, if anything, a larger degree of residual pancreatic parenchyma but failed to respond to conservative measures, required surgery and subsequently died (Figure 6b). Both scans revealed severe changes in the pancreas and surrounding tissues but there were no specific features on either scan which indicated that one patient would do poorly and the other well. This illustrates the limitations of CT in the management of patients with severe acute pancreatitis and emphasises the need for close liaison between clinician and radiologist during the course of this difficult illness.

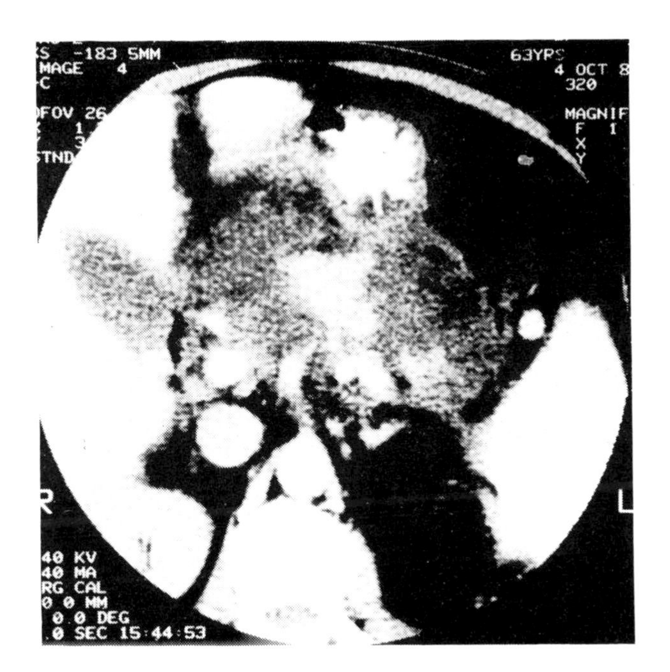

Figure 6b

Conclusion

We in Leeds feel that high dose dynamic CT can give an accurate indication of the existance and extent of pancreatic necrosis. The demonstration of necrosis does not itself indicate surgery, but should surgery be required, the CT images provide the surgeon with a'road map' to help plan his approach and guide finger dissection.

DISCUSSION

CT SCANNING

Shorvon: I agree that the presence of CT detected pancreatic necrosis is not always an indication for surgery. Recently five patients with "CT necrotising pancreatitis" did not undergo surgery. Only one patient died in that group. We have treated infected pseudocysts percutaneously, largely under CT direction, inserting increasingly larger drains using antibiotic cover and intensive care management.Ultrasound can be used in acute pancreatitis to follow fluid collections quite carefully, but CT is often necessary to avoid bowel during drainage procedures. Ultrasound in the very acute phase is often unsatisfactory as it cannot distinguish an inflammatory mass from a necrotic one and suboptimal views are often obtained. Allan's point on peripheral pancreatitis was interesting. A German paper (1) reported an ERCP study on acute pancreatitis and distinguished two types of patients. In one the duct system was essentially filled throughout with no leakage, and in the other the duct system was disrupted or leaking. The former only required debridement of peripheral necrotic tissue at surgery as opposed to pancreactic resection that was usually required in the rest. The former presumably relate to the group who have central preservation of pancreatic tissue with peripheral necrosis.

Finally, I would like to support the view that CT scanning is important for these patients as it indicates pancreatic necrosis and gives information on impending complications. It should become a important part of any prognostic assessment, but to be so usefully, it will need to be undertaken by those with a special interest. It requries high contrast dose infusion techniques in rapid scanning modes.

McMahon: In those patients whose condition takes a malignant course, there appear to be two principal determinants: central necrosis with interruption of the duct system and inhibition of pancreatic juice drainage, and infection. In Britain we are now in a position to weigh the importance of these factors in a prospective and worthwhile manner. The Americans, Gerzof et al,(2) and Hiatt (3) showed that fine needle aspiration of pancreatic collections is safe and showed that approximately 50-60% are infected. Their work has led to a consensus view in the United States that if you find infection you must operate or at least ensure that drainage by percutaneous techniques is complete. We are in a position however, to determine the importance of infection to the clinical course of pancreatic necrosis and to find out if the presence of infection can explain the apparant lack of correlation between CT appearances and the progress of the patient.

Trapnell: Are you then saying that a fine needle aspirate should be an additional arm of our prognostic investigation?

McMahon: Yes. It does not have a routine place in clinical management yet,but it may well become routine if it's value can be established and it's safety confirmed.

Imrie: Pat Freeney in Seattle has just published work in the American radiological literature explaining how they have been inserting large drains into the area of sepsis without surgical intervention. I am sure this area should become one of shared responsibilty between interventional radiology and surgery, loculated areas of sepsis to be dealt with by the radiologist, and the non-loculated, more profuse septic problem requiring wide debridement and multiple drains by the surgeon. Beger in Germany and Bradley in Atlanta are achieving almost 90% survival rates with these techniques. In this country figures around 60% are common.

Neoptolemos: I think we are too readily accepting statements being made about CT, necrosis and pancreatitis. We do not know the natural history of hypoperfusion of the pancreas with contrast enhanced CT. What does decreased enhancement mean? You cannot on the one hand say, "We are showing necrosis on CT," and on the other hand report the patient making a complete and total recovery.
It may be possible to provide part of the answer with a prospective randomised trial, although there would be considerable logistical problems in trying to do so.

Taylor: I am intrigued by this peripheral rim of necrosis. Do you see this in just the alcoholic pancreatitis or gallstone pancreatitis as well?

Chalmers: In both.

Taylor: Whatever aetiology you favour for gallstone associated pancreatitis, would you not expect the severe necrosis to be found in the central part of the pancreas?

Trapnell: The peripancreatic tissue is far more sensitive to digestion than the gland, as it is less well perfused. Presumably this rim tissue is the so-called "peripancreatic slough", reported at operation over many years.

Russell: The condition of the duct is the key to the whole process of the disease. It is a progressive disease, but if the duct is intact, the patient is able to recover, no matter what the necrosis looks like on the CT scan. I very much go along with Freeney's work where he aims to keep the surgeon out of the abdomen. If you drain the majority of these collections percutaneously, and use small drains rather than large ones that lead to fistulation , there will be an improvement in results. I think that infecton too can resolve spontaneously by natural fistulation, and so I believe one can continue with conservative management and I would suggest this as an alternative to rapid operative intervention.

Chalmers: In our experience small drains will not function with severely necrotic peripancreatic tissue.

Shorvon: In that case change to bigger catheters and multiple drains if necessary.

PATHOGENESIS: Is infection primary or secondary?

Imrie: I feel that infection is not primary for several reasons. If bacteria were instrumental in the initial pathogenesis of this process, it is difficult to understand how 40% of patients with severe pancreatitis are found to have a sterile necrotic mass. I would also contest that infected necrosis, when it occurs, starts from the earliest point. Even Berger's group detected infected necrosis only by Day 4 or 5. The evidence may change with more CT guided needle aspiration, but I have the impression that infection occurs later in the process,not ab initio.

Trapnell : There are two studies that show that the use of antibiotics does not alter prognosis.

Jones: It is generally accepted that infection, primary or secondary, is present in those people that die from pancreatitis and is the major cause of death in this situation. The two trials mentioned earlier were in alcoholic patients with an overall low mortality, were retrospective, and used first generation antibiotics including Tetracyline, which itself has been incriminated as a cause of pancreatitis. I feel that this is an area which ought to be explored further with the early selection of patients with severe pancreatitis and aggressive treatment with broader spectrum agents covering the organisms mentioned in previous discussion and would be hopeful that this would reduce the mortality. I believe it might at least prevent early sepsis and if patients did require surgical intervention for infection, they would be in a more stable condition to survive it.

Trapnell: Does this view have any support? Is this something that the Pancreatic Society would want to take up?

Neoptolemos: We must make a distinction between bacteria as triggers of acute pancreatitis and bacteria contributing to the pathogenesis and final outcome. I see no reason why bacterial amidases should not trigger acute pancreatitis, but to extend this and say that they cause infection does not necessarily follow. We know that bacteria are involved in a high proportion of cases of severe pancreatic necrosis and I think most people use antibiotics routinely, as part of the overall management.

Jones: There is a difference of opinion there. It has been discussed at the Pancreatic Society meetings before and I am not sure that everybody uses antibiotics in this way.

Imrie: It would be difficult to set up a study in the gallstone group as few clinicians suspect or prove aetiology sufficiently early. I think it might be possible to mount a controlled study in the alcohol group, providing it took place North of the Wash.

McMahon : I do not give antibiotics unless cholangitis or cholecystitis is a possibility; not if the liver function tests are descending, yes, if they are ascending.

Jones: I give them to all patients with pancreatitis at the time of diagnosis and stop them if the prognostic indicators shows that the patient does not fall within the severe group after 48 hours. I use Pipril with Fluclox-icillin or in patients with Penicillin allergies, a 3rd generation Cephalosporin with Gentamicin.

Leese: A multicentre study in Rotterdam is taking this one step further, both antibiotic usage and gut irrigation are being randomised. The aggressive gut lavage is intended to reduce the gut flora.

Keynes: How does secondary infection occur?

Russell: The supporters of the oxygen free radical theory believe that in states of shock there is a loss of the mucosal barrier of the bowel. A migration across the bowel wall into the peritoneal fluid of bacteria can be shown.

DETECTION OF THE HIGH RISK PATIENT

Keynes: Have the trypsinogen activated peptide levels been related to those of serum amylase, which is also elevated.

Imrie: Yes, and it is not useful. 20% of the patients on admission to hospital have a rising serum amylase. This is not generally appreciated, most text books teach that amylase is maximal at admission.

Keynes : Don't trypsinogen activation peptide levels go on rising in this 48 hours?

Imrie: The activation of trypsinogen is an early marker; it distinguishes those with mild and severe disease, and correlates well with the clinical outcome of the disease. It is conceptually very different to measurements of inactive enzymes.

IDIOPATHIC PANCREATITIS

Imrie: This group of patients demands a great deal more study. It causes me much concern, and yet it is a group of patients who are conveniently forgotten in the analysis of nearly every prospective study. I cannot find a single study in which the so-called idiopathic group does not have maximal mortality rates. They tend to be the oldest group of patients and whether they have an ischaemic pancreatitis or whether they have microlithiasis, one does not really know.

Larvin: Based on my experiences around the Yorkshire region, I wonder whether, because these older patients are not usually subjected to post-mortem, and they die on the second or third day before they have had an ultrasound, we are missing gallstones in that group and they are not really idiopathic at all.

Russell: I believe that many patients who have pancreatitis attributed to gallstones or alcohol do not have such an aetiology at all. I think that we are not looking closely enough at the pathology. When studied carefully quite bizarre things are found in their pancreases, including small duodenal cysts, and pancreatic tumours.

Trapnell: Unfortunately the number of autopsies that are being performed in our hospitals is diminishing rapidly. 30 years ago in Bristol a great deal of post-mortem data was available. We do not have access to that these days. Maybe CT and ultrasound will give other information to us. Also we must not ignore the patients who die of pancreatitis secondary to hypothermia, carbon monoxide poisoning, collagen diseases and eclampsia. These conditions are important when considering the whole spectrum of pathology in this condition. Mortality rates have not changed and I agree with Mr Russell's point that we should consider the pathological evidence more closeley.

McMahon: Interesting data has been obtained by sieving faeces and it was shown that in Leeds a concerted hunt for gallstones could cut the idiopathic group down to half the size. I feel that many of these patients have gallstones.

Trapnell: Mr Imrie, how do you think the idiopathic group should be tackled?

Imrie: I am sure that the efforts of a dedicated individual for as a short period as two years in one hospital, with modern technology, and not so modern technology including faecal sieving, might well eliminate this idiopathic group or make it so small that it could almost be discounted, and not run at the level of 20% seen in many of the prospective multicentre studies.

Trapnell: Where does that leave your comment that it has a higher mortality?

Imrie : As pointed out, the patients tend to be older, and they do not have post-mortems. It may be simply a function of age, but it may be that the therapy is not so good in these patients, and that doctors have not pushed sufficiently hard for post-mortems for various reasons.

References

1. Gebhardt C. Diagnostic procedures in pancreatic disease. Editors P Malferheiner and H Ditchuneit, Springer Verlag Berlin (1985), pages 49-53
2. Gerzof SG, Johnson WC, Robbins AH, Spechler SJ, Nabseth DC. Percutaneous drainage of infected pancreatic pseudocysts. *Arch Surg* 1984; 119: 888-93.
3. Hiatt JR, Fink AS, King W, Pitt HA. Percutaneous aspiration of peripancreatic fluid collection, a safe method to detect infection. *Surg* 1987;101: 523-30.

THE FUTURE OF MEDICAL TREATMENT OF ACUTE PANCREATITIS.

Dr P R Salmon
Consultant Gastroenterologist
Harley House
London

Introduction

The term acute pancreatitis covers a whole spectrum of pathological changes and processes in the pancreas and other organ systems which together carry a mortality of about 10%. The remaining cases are largely self limiting and the patients recover fully. The mortality associated with acute pancreatitis has fallen from about 25% to 10% or less over the past 25 years, largely as a result of better supportive care. Our understanding of the pathogenesis of acute pancreatitis and the detection of those cases that are likely to do badly and therefore require intensive treatment falls far short of the ideal.

Identification of the high risk case

Prognostic grading systems have been discussed in detail by Imrie but at best they are a useful guide, and at worst fail to discriminate between the potentially fatal case and the one that will recover fully regardless of treatment. Ranson, Rifkind, et al (1) were the first to discuss prognostic signs fully, and in a retrospective study they analysed the prognostic value of 43 objective measurements obtained within 48 hours of hospital admission in patients with acute pancreatitis. They identified 11 early prognostic signs of which 5 were obtained at the time of admission and 6 obtained during the ensuing 48 hours. When applied prospectively in a series of 200 cases of acute pancreatitis, 162 patients had less than three of the 11 criteria, and only one patient (0.6%) developed a major complication and died. On the other hand, 24/38 patients (63%) with three or more prognostic signs became severely ill or died. On this basis acute pancreatitis was classified as mild if less than three prognostic signs were present, and severe if three or more signs were positive. In a further larger study (450 cases of acute pancreatitis) Ranson and Spencer (2) showed a mortality rate of 1% for those with less than three prognostic signs, 16% with three to four prognostic signs, 40% with five

	No of prognostic signs			
	0-2	3-4	5-6	7-8
No of patients	347	67	30	6
Mortality No,(%)	3(0.9)	11(16)	12(40)	6(100)
No(%)died or in ICU	13(3.7)	27(40)	28(93)	6(100)

Table 1. Prognostic signs in acute pancreatitis and mortality(2)

to six prognostic signs, and 100% with seven or more prognostic signs (Table 1).

Since the first grading system was developed there have been numerous refinements including for example the inclusion of physical signs as well as laboratory findings at the time of admission or within 48 hours (3), the presence of methaemalbumin as an adverse prognostic marker (4), and the use of peritoneal lavage to assess the severity of acute pancreatitis (5). Imrie and others have done much work on blood measurements as prognostic markers, including measurement of fibrinogen, LDH, and latterly C-reactive protein. The problem of the relatively large proportion of cases of acute pancreatitis who do not readily fall into the severe pancreatitis group remains however, and reflects our lack of precise knowledge of the pathogenesis of acute pancreatitis.

NON-OPERATIVE MANAGEMENT.

The initial management of acute pancreatitis is supportive and non-operative and is based on the premise that acute pancreatitis is based on pancreatic hypersecretion in the presence of ductal obstruction (at the ampulla of Vater or elsewhere), resulting in extravasation of activated enzymes into the gland parenchyma. With this theory initiation of acute pancreatitis lies in the interstitial space. For a number of reasons this hypothesis is likely to be incorrect. In the first place specific measures to suppress pancreatic secretion have no beneficial effect on the prognosis of acute pancreatitis.

Supportive Care

General supportive measures are however fundamental in the management of acute pancreatitis:

1. Intravascular fluid management.

Early replacement and maintenance of adequate intravascular volume is important and should take the form of early, aggressive volume resuscitation in order to maintain tissue perfusion, and in particular the pancreatic microcirculation. The volumes required vary but may be as much as 8 L. of fluid within 24 hours in severe cases. Heart rate, blood pressure and urine output should be used to assess the adequacy of replacement with urinary catheterization using a urimeter drainage bag to ensure that the output is at least 30 ml/hr, and in severe cases a central venous pressure line to assess right and left ventricular filling pressures may be required. Maintenance of plasma colloid osmotic pressure is of paramount importance. Albumin infusions have been used but crystalloid resuscitation may be just as good. It should be remembered that Dextran 70 can cause acute renal failure and that plasma proteins can transmit hepatitis or HIV. Fresh frozen plasma (3 units daily) will provide antitrypsin and alpha -2 - macroglobulin. It should be remembered that the patient with severe pancreatitis may look deceptively well.

2. Analgesia.

Pain relief may be an important aspect of acute pancreatitis management. Whilst in theory pethidine is preferable to morphine since the latter can cause spasm of the sphincter of Oddi, a combination of morphine (15 mg.) and cyclizine (10 mg.) is usually effective. Epidural anaesthesia and splanchnic block as an alternative, in order to avoid sphincter of Oddi spasm and to improve pancreatic micro circulation have not gained widespread acceptance.

3. Nuritional support.

Oral intake should be greatly reduced or abolished in the early management of acute pancreatis if for no other reason that it satisfies one of the current concepts (albeit probably incorrect), viz. suppression of pancreatic secretion, in the management of acute pancreatitis. However there may be a persistent paralytic ileus or pain in association with a pancreatic inflammatory mass which precludes oral intake, and for these reasons parenteral nutrition is an important aspect of early management in severe acute pancreatitis. Goodgame and Fischer (6) showed that TPN had no specific beneficial effect on the pathophysiology of acute pancreatitis but was a useful adjunctive measure.

4. Antibiotics.

Prophylactic antibiotics have been used in acute pancreatitis. There is no good evidence however that the routine use of antibiotics is of value in patients with mild or moderately severe acute pancreatitis. A randomized prospective study from The Johns Hopkins Hospital (7) demonstrated this point. (Table 2)

	Antibiotics	No antibiotics
No of patients	45	47
Amylase elevation (days)	2	2
Fever(days)	3	3
Hospitalization(days)	9	12
Septic complications	5	6

Table 2. Prophylactic antibiotics in acute pancreatitis . (7)

5. Respiratory support

Respiratory complications are well recognized features of acute pancreatitis having been studied by McKenna et al (8), and by Imrie et al (9). They occur in 15-55% of cases and include pleural effusions, atelectasis, pneumonia, and acute respiratory insufficiency. Arterial hypoxaemia is a further important feature which may indicate occult respiratory insufficiency. Routine arterial blood gas estimations every 12 hours are recommended for all cases of severe acute pancreatitis. Supplemental oxygen should be given to those cases with an arterial PaO_2 of less than 70 mm Hg.

6. Peritoneal dialysis.

Peritoneal dialysis has been employed since 1965 for the treatment of severe acute pancreatitis. (10) The therapeutic efficacy is presumably due to the removal of potentially toxic biologically active compounds that are found in peritoneal exudate in acute pancreatitis. These include phospholipase A, trypsinogen, vasoactive kinins, and prostaglandins. Whilst the literature is conflicting there is a place for peritoneal lavage in the early course of severe acute pancreatitis. Since there is usually significant bowel distention in acute pancreatitis insertion of the peritoneal dialysis catheter is preferably placed by an open technique (small surgical incision). Isotonic dialysis solution containing 15 G/L glucose is usually employed, whilst heparin (1,000 USP), ampicillin (250 mg), and potassium (8 mEq) are added to each 2 L of dialysate. Since the infusion of dialysate may restrict diaphragm movements and aggravate occult or overt respiratory insufficiency, careful monitoring of blood gases is mandatory. Blood glucose levels should also be carefully monitored during peritoneal dialysis.

Suppression of Pancreatic Secretion.

Measures to suppress pancreatic secretion as mentioned are all based on the belief that the pathogenesis of acute pancreatitis involves on the one hand pancreatic hypersecretion and on the other pancreatic ductal obstruction. Almost without exception these measures are ineffective in improving the prognosis of acute pancreatitis, putting the above hypothesis severely to the test.

1. Nasogastric suction

Whilst nasogastric suction has been considered standard therapy in acute pancreatitis for many years, by means of reducing acid-induced secretin release from the duodenum, no beneficial effect of routine nasogastric suction has been demonstrated. At least nine randomized controlled trials have failed to show an improvement of mortality or prognosis. The only indication for its use in acute pancreatitis is with persistent vomiting, gastric distention and to reduce aspiration in confused patients.

2. Gastric hyposecretory drugs

The use of histamine 2 receptor antagonists (H2RA) as a means of inhibiting gastric acid secretion and therefore acid mediated duodenal secretin-release, is rational but nevertheless has not been shown to be beneficial in patients with acute pancreatitis. A number of studies from the Johns Hopkins Hospital (11) failed to show any value of cimetidine in patients with acute pancreatitis. The use of atropine is also time honoured but does not appear to have any benefit. The rationale includes its use as a hyposecretory agent but also includes inhibition of vagally medicated pancreatic secretion, and relaxation of the sphincter of Oddi. Its use, as with other anticholinergic agents, should now cease in acute pancreatitis.

3. Glucagon

Glucagon suppresses both the volume and enzyme secretion of the stimulated pancreas and also inhibits gastric secretion. Glucagon also decreased mortality when administered early in experimental pancreatitis. (12) Early uncontrolled data was encouraging when glucagon was used in acute pancreatitis but prospective randomized trials have failed to show a benefit .(13)

4. Calcitonin

Calcitonin reduces pancreatic enzyme secretion following exocrine stimulation with various secretogogues, and also reduces pentagastrin-stimulated gastric acid secretion. A number of studies have demonstrated significant reduction of pain and also amylase levels in acute pancreatitis but none have demonstrated any reduction in mortality.

5. Somatostatin

Somatostatin has a similar action to calcitonin on pancreatic and gastric secretion. Once again the results of controlled trials have failed to substantiate the optimistic results of earlier uncontrolled studies.(14)

Inhibition of pancreatic enzymes

This is a further measure that in theory should be of value in acute pancreatitis. A number of specific enzyme inhibitors are available and have been studied.

1. Aprotinin

Aprotinin is a potent inhibitor of the proteolytic enzymes trypsin, chymotrypsin, and kallikrein. Controlled trials have however failed to show in man, that aprotinin either improves the course or the mortality of acute pancreatitis. (15)

2. Antifibrinolytics

Epsilon-aminocaproic acid (EACA) and p-aminomethylbenzoic acid (PAMBA) inhibit plasmin and trypsin but have not been shown to have a beneficial effect in acute pancreatitis. (16)

3. Phospholipase A- inhibitors

Phospholipase-A produces a highly toxic substance, lysolecithin from lecithin, so that inhibition of phospholipase-A would appear to be of value in acute pancreatitis. Calcium disodium editate (Ca Na_2 EDTA) has however not been shown to alter the prognosis or mortality of acute pancreatitis.

Intracellular Theory

The disappointing results from so many theoretically successful measures leaves the "ductal hypertension" theory of acute pancreatitis in serious doubt. For this reason and because pancreatitis is so complex, and because the pancreas is relatively inaccessible to both clinical and experimental observations, a number of animal models have been developed. Some of these models have now for the first time pointed strongly to defects within the pancreatic acinar cell in acute pancreatitis. Deranged intracellular transport of secretory proteins appears to be the primary lesion. In two important animal models (The choline deficient ethionine supplemented diet - CDE diet, and the secretogogue induced pancreatitis model) protein synthesis and intracellular transport to the Golgi complex remained normal but the secretion of digestive enzymes was blocked. Digestive enzymes remained in large vacuoles containing lysosomal hydrolases that were capable of activating trypsinogen. Colocalization of digestive enzymes and lysosomal hydrolases could in theory result in activation of digestive enzymes resulting in release of activated enzymes into the acinar cell cytoplasm. There are obviously many questions still to be answered but the intracellular theory of acute pancreatitis has much to commend it currently. As far as medical management of acute pancreatitis is concerned with respect to the intracellular theory, a complete change of thinking must take place. We must now for example begin to think about treatment aimed at restoring normal patterns of intracellular transport as well as drugs that block activation of enzymes within the acinar cell and drugs that block lysosomal hydrolases such as cathepsin-B.

References

1. Ranson JH, Rifkind KM, Roses DF, et al. Prognostic signs and the role of operative management in acute pancreatitis. *Surg Gynecol Obstet* 1974; 139 (i) : 69-81.
2. Ranson JH and Spencer FC. The role of peritoneal lavage in severe acute pancreatitis. Ann Surg 1978; 187 (5): 565-575.
3. Jacobs ML, Dagett WM, Cirvette JM et al. Acute pancreatitis: analysis of factors influencing survival. *Ann Surg* 1977; 185 (i): 43-51.
4. Lankisch P, Koop H, Otto J et al. Evaluation of methaemalbumin in acute pancretitis. *Scand J. Gastroenterol* 1978; 13 (8):975-978.
5. McMahon MJ, Playforth MJ, Pickford IR. A comparative study of methods for the prediction of severity of attacks of acute pancreatitis. *Br J Surg* 1980; 67 (i): 22-25.
6. Goodgame JT, Fischer JE. Parenteral nutrition in the treatment of acute pancreatitis: effect on complications and mortality. *Ann Surg* 1977; 186 (5): 651-658.
7. Howes R, Zuldema GD, Cameron JL. Evaluation of prophylactic antibiotics in acute pancreatitis. *J Surg Res* 1975; 18 (2): 197-200.
8. McKenna JM, Chandrasekhar AJ, Skorton D et al. The pleuropulmonary complications of pancreatitis. *Chest* 1977; 71 (2): 197-204.
9. Imrie CW, Ferguson JC, Murphy D, et al. Arterial hypoxia in acute pancreatitis. *Br J Surg* 1977; 64 (3): 185-188.
10. Wall AJ. Peritoneal dialysis in the treatment of severe acute pancreatitis. *Med J Aust* 1965; 2 (7): 281-283.
11. Broe PJ, Zinner MJ, Cameron JL. A clinical trial of cimetidine in acute pancreatitis. *Surg Gynecol Obstet* 1982; 154 (i): 13-16.
12. Waterworth MW, Barbezat GO, Hickman R et al. A controlled trial of glucagon in experimental pancreatitis. *Br J Surg* 1976; 63 (8): 617-620.
13. Medical Research Council: Multicentre trial of glucagon and aprotinin: Death from acute pancreatitis. *Lancet* 1977; 2: 623-635.
14. Usadel KH, Leuschner U, Uberla KK. Treatment of acute pancreatitis with somatostatin: a multi-center double blind trial. *N Engl J Med* 1980; 303: 999-1000.
15. Imrie CW, Benjamin IS, Ferguson JC et al. A single-center double -blind trial of Trasylol therapy in primary acute pancreatitis. *Br J Surg* 1978; 65 (5): 337-341.
16. Konttinen YP. Epsilon-aminocaproic acid in treatment of acute pancreatitis. *Scand J Gastroenterol* 1971; 6 (8): 715-718.

Suggested Reading:
Steer ML, Meldolesi J. "The cell biology of experimental pancreatitis" New Engl J Med 1987: 316; 144-150

THE ROLE OF ENDOSCOPIC SPHINCTEROTOMY AND SURGERY IN THE TREATMENT OF ACUTE GALLSTONE PANCREATITIS

Mr J P Neoptolemos
Senior Lecturer
Department of Surgery
University of Birmingham

Introduction

Ambrose Pare probably provided the first clear description of acute pancreatitis in 1579 (1) and he drew notice to the importance of dietary factors in its aetiology. Historically, the pancreas (all meat) does not appear to have excited much interest amongst physicians. Only sporadic mention was made of acute pancreatitis until Reginald Fitz presented the first major collected series involving 53 cases to the New York Pathological Society in 1889. (2)

In 1901, Eugene Opie was able to collect 32 cases of acute pancreatitis in which gallstones were also present and be emphasised a causal relationship. (3) In a subsequent paper in the same year, (4) he proposed the "common channel" theory which could explain how a stone impacted at the ampulla of Vater enabled bile to reflux into the pancreatic duct. This incorporated the work of Claude Bernard who showed in 1856 that pancreatitis could be induced by bile injected into the pancreatic duct (5) and of Lancereaux who proposed the bile reflux theory in human acute pancreatitis. (6)

These theoretical studies led to important practical innovations. The two giants of surgery practising at this time, William Mayo and Sir Berkeley Moynihan, became great advocates of urgent surgical intervention, laying emphasis on decompression of the biliary tree in the presence of jaundice and/or gallstones. (7,8) The results of anatomical studies, however, soon questioned the common channel theory. (9) The advent of improved means of supportive care (10), and the often poor results of surgery, led to a more conservative approach.

Although Glenn (11) and Frey, (12) amongst others, attempted to push the pendulum back again in the 1950's and 1960's, the theoretical field remained sterile. Two papers were published in 1974, however, which were to be of enormous significance. The first paper, by Ranson from New York, showed that the likely outcome of an acute attack of pancreatitis could be predicted_by using objective clinical and biochemical criteria at the time of admission. (13) These criteria and the modification(s) proposed by Imrie and the Glasgow group, (14-16) have become widely established. The second paper was that of Acosta and Ledesma from Argentina which showed that virtually all patients with acute gallstone pancreatitis pass stones into the faeces, (17) It was proposed that bile refluxed into the pancreatic duct (PD) because of oedema at the ampulla of Vater. Alternatively, it has been proposed that the passage of a stone may cause the ampulla of Vater to gape, allowing reflux of activated duodenal enzymes. (18)

The work of Acosta and Ledesma subsequently received confirmation. (19,20) Paradoxically, this led some to advocate aggressive surgical biliary decompression (21-24) and others to advocate a more conservative approach. (15,25-28)These studies floundered because of inadequately controlled groups, inadequate use of prognostic criteria or both. Endoscopic retrograde cholangiopancreatography (ERCP) and endoscopic sphincterotomy (ES) with common bile duct (CBD) stone extraction seemed attractive (29-33) compared to surgical biliary decompression but these studies too suffered from identical drawbacks.

At the centre of the controversy lay perhaps not so much the absence of a cohesive theory of biliary pancreatitis, but the rejection of seemingly conflicting theories. In 1658 Gassendi had argued that theories were not to be put up on the pulpit to be judged as true or false, indeed they could not be so considered. Rather they were to be judged as successful or unsuccessful as intruments by which knowledge could be made orderly and penetrating. (34) To paraphrase Plato, (35) it is absurd to devote all our energies to securing the greatest possible precision and clarity in matters of little consequence, and not to demand the highest pracision in the most important thing(s) of all. In the context of biliary pancreatitis, the central question is "What is the precise relationship between common bile duct stones and the natural history of acute pancreatitis". The two developments which have made it possible to get closer to answering this question have been ERCP and prognostic criteria of severity.

The corollary to this has now been the establishment of endoscopic sphincterotomy as part of the treatment of gallstone pancreatitis. But what of the patient who has not benefitted from such an approach and has developed extensive necrotizing pancreatitis? In 1886 Senn had suggested "that timely removal of the necrosed (pancreas) by surgical interference would add to the chances of recovery".(36)

The role of surgical resection or sequestrectomy has been as controversial as the role of biliary decompression ever since. As in the case of ERCP, two other technological advances have made a significant impact on this particular aspect of pancreatitis. These are computerised tomography (CT) and interventional radiology. Although this chapter will largly concentrate on the particular problem of gallstones in acute pancreatitis, modern surgical approaches to necrotising pancreatitis will also be discussed.

URGENT DETECTION OF GALLSTONES IN ACUTE PANCREATITIS

From a pragmatic point of view, it is essential to be able to detect gallstones in patients with acute pancreatitis before embarking on ERCP, because of potential hazards.

It had been found previously that acute cholecystitis was sometimes a feature of patients with acute pancreatitis who had undergone an urgent* laparotomy. (37) The introduction of radionuclide biliary scanning in the mid 1970's offered the opportunity to examine the relationship between the biliary tree and acute pancreatitis early on in an attack. Although the finding of gallbladder non-filling (a "positive" result) was more common in acute biliary pancreatitis, it could not be used to differentiate biliary from non biliary pancreatitis.(38) A subsequent expanded series reached identical conclusions. (39)

The failure of gallbladder filling in the biliary group could be due to oedema from recent stone passage through the cystic duct, but in both groups could be due to stasis of bile in the gallbladder as occurs, say, after laparotomy, (40) or due to oedema of the cystic duct secondary to retrograde lymphangitis.(41) The time taken for the isotope to enter the small bowel, perhaps prolonged due to stones in or oedema of, the ampulla of Vater also failed to differentiate between gallstone and non-gallstone pancreatitis.(39)

Some studies have reported radionucleptide biliary scanning to be of value in diagnosing acute biliary pancreatitis, (42-45) but others have supported our findings. (46-49) Disappointingly, one authority continues to recommend this investigation in this situation.(50)

In 1978, McKay and colleagues from Glasgow reported that urgent ultrasonography (US) in acute pancreatitis had a 58% sensitivity with 5% false positives, but 31% of investigations were not useful.(51) Our own studies using updated equipment achieved better results: a sensitivity of 62% and no false positives.(39) Re-scanning later during the same admission improved the sensitivity to 78% which was useful for planning early cholecystectomy. The main difficulty in both these studies was masking of the gallbladder in the first 72 hours by overlying gas due to the ileus of pancreatitis. The introduction of even more advanced ultrasound equipment is unlikely to improve this situation.

The biochemical prediction of gallstones in acute pancreatitis is now established, but all the methods proposed result in a significant proportion of false negatives.(52-56) The use of relatively high cut-off points (bilirubin >55 μmol/l, alkaline phosphatase >400 iu/l and alanine transaminase >170 iu/l) gives a low sensitivity, but could be combined with US to provide an overall sensitivity of 80% without false positives.(39) We used this approach to explore the use of ERCP in acute pancreatitis, and to design the first prospective randomized trial of ERCP ± ES versus conventional treatment in acute pancreatitis due to suspected gallstones.(57)

Although computerised axial tomography has been shown to have a reasonably good sensitivity in gallstone detection in the non-urgent situation,(58) our own studies in over 100 patients with acute pancreatitis found a sensitivity of only 34%.(59)

*Footnote: The terms urgent, early, delayed and late are used to describe investigations or treatment, undertaken at <72 hours, 3-30 days, 1-6 months and >6 months respectively from the first day of the attack.

EFFECTS OF PERSISTING COMMON BILE DUCT STONES

Relationship to outcome

Over a ten year period 100 patients with acute pancreatitis unequivocally due to gallstones had an ERCP during the same admission.(60) Fifty-five patients had an urgent ERCP and 45 patients had an early ERCP. Complications occured in 19 patients, including two deaths (Table 1).

The overall incidence of CBD stones was 37%; incidence was greater in those with predicted severs (PS) than in those with predicted mild (PM)

Complications	Total
Pseudocysts	4
Pancreatic necrosis	4 (2†)
Pancreatic asbscess	4 (1†)
Peri-pancreatic abscess	3(1†)
Liver abscess	1
Pseudo-obstruction	1
Respiratory failure	5(1†)
Multisystem failure	1(†)
DIC	1
Lumbar osteitis	1
Empyema of gallbladder	1
Number of patients with complications	19
Number of deaths	2

†Complications associated with death

TABLE 1 Complications in 100 patients with gallstone associated pancreatitis undergoing ERCP ± ES during the same admissions (n = 100)

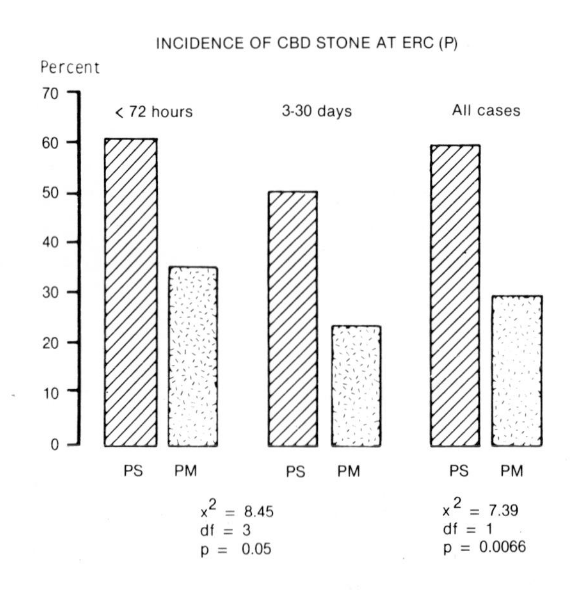

Fig. 1 Relative incidence of common bile duct (CBD) stones in relation to urgent (<72 hours) or early (3-30 days) ERCP and predicted severity of the attack. PS = predicted severe; PM = predicted mild.

attacks and was, highest in those with PS attacks during the first 72 hours (Fig.1).

The incidence of complications was, as anticipated, greater in those with PS attacks but was also significantly greater in those with persisting CBD stones (Fig. 2), a new finding. Furthermore, the presence of CBD stones determined severity more than conventional predictive factors: thus patients with PM attacks and CBD stones had more complications than those with PS attacks and no CBD stones (Fig. 3).

We have recently reported that the association between acute cholangitis and pancreatitis is much commoner than previouly considered. (61) This association was well recognised by surgeons in the eary part of this century, but has only received sporadic mention since. (62-65) In the present series, 23 of the 100 patients had acute cholangitis; 13 of 38 patients (34%) with PS attacks had acute cholangitis compared with 10 of 62 patients with PM attacks (16%; $X^2 = 4.35$, df = 1, p = 0.0366). Fifteen of these patients (65%) had CBD stones: 10 of the 13 with PS attacks (77%) and five of the 10 with PM attacks (50%). This corroborates the importance of persisting CBD stones, as such patients have a higher incidence of pancreatic complications compared to those with acute pancreatitis alone. (66)

Obstruction of the common bile duct and pancreatic duct

Patients with gallstone pancreatits have a wider CBD than those with non-biliary pancreatitis (60), whilst those with gallstone pancreatitis and CBD stones have a wider CBD than those without stones. (60) We have however, recently demonstrated a correlation between CBD diameter and age irrespective of underlying pathology (unpublished) and as patients with CBD stones were older, their wider CBD might be due to this alone. Using analysis of covariance to control for age, however, a continuing increase in CBD diameter in patients with CBD stones was revealed. (60)

Armstrong et al in a study of operative cholangiography, showed that-patients with gallstone pancreatitis had a greater pancreatic duct (PD) (as shown on the reflux pancreatogram) than those with gallstones but no pancreatitis.(67) Surprisingly, in our studies using ERCP the PD did not differ significantly when all cases with and without CBD stones were compared. This finding, however, was apparent rather than real (60) for the following reasons. Analysis of the patients with PM attacks revealed a wider PD in those with CBD stones (4.27 + 1.24 mm) than in those without CBD stones (3.41 + 1.09 mm; $p<0.05$). Filling of the PD occurred in 82% of patients with PM attacks, irrespective of the presence of CBD stones; in

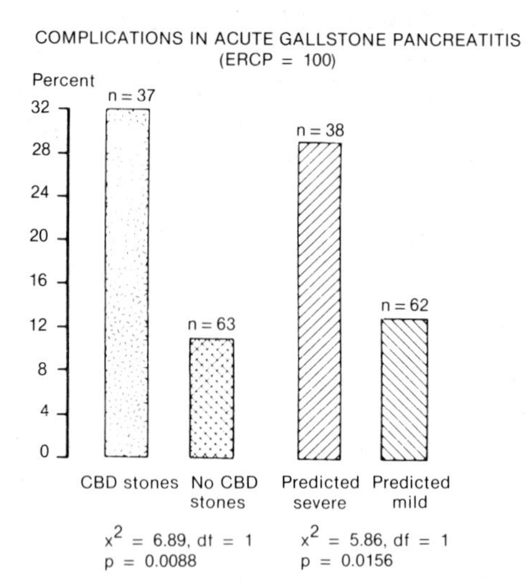

Fig 2 Actual complications developing in acute gallstone pancreatitis comparing those with and without common bile duct (CBD) stones (LEFT) and predicted severity of the attack (RIGHT).

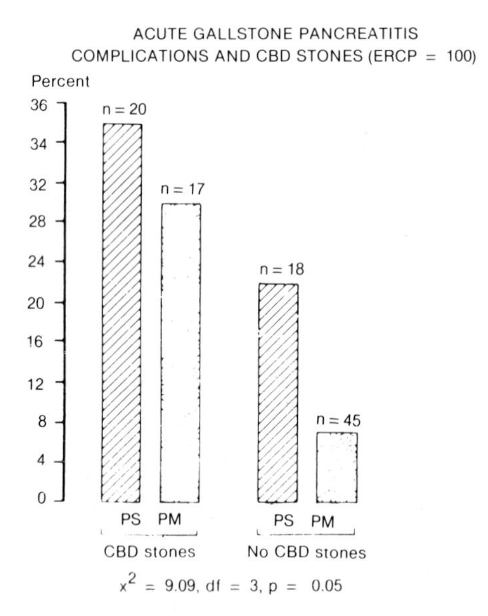

Fig. 3 Actual complications developing in acute gallstone pancreatitis when considering presence or absence of common bile duct (CBD) stones in combination with predicted severity of the attack. PS = predicted severe; PM = predicted mild.

patients with PS attacks, however, PD filling occured in only 50% of those with CBD stones compared to 95% in those without CBD stones ($p<0.01$). The incidence of successful cholangiography at ERC(P) was similar in all groups (80% - 100%). This suggests obstruction of the PD by persisting CBD stones which are much more frequent in severe cases.

Two further findings support combined CBD and PD obstruction(60).Significant positive correlations were observed between CBD and PD diameters, even after correction for age,(60), and between the admission serum bilirubin and CBD diameter. An elevated admission serum transaninase indicates transient gallstone migration, but raised serum bilirubin indicates persisting CBD stones.(55,68) The correlationn between admission serum bilirubin and PD diameter was therefore, the final piece of evidence supporting our contention that PD obstruction occurs in acute gallstone pancreatitis.

THE DETECTION OF COMMON BILE DUCT STONES

It should now be apparent that patients with gallstones and PS attacks are likely to have CBD stones. All such patients should be seriously considered for ERC(P) to confirm this, and our overall results including patients without gallstones, demonstrate that this approach is relatively safe(60) if undertaken by an experienced endoscopist.

The indication for ERCP may be considerably enhanced by the finding on admission of a serum bilirubin of >40 µmol/1. Our original experience(68) has now been expanded to the current series of 100 patients with biliary pancreatitis and 31 patients with non-biliary pancreatitis, all undergoing urgent or early ERCP.(60) The results showed that with a bilirubin > 40 µmol/1, over 78% of patients with CBD stones were detected, with a specificity of 77%. With a bilirubin <40 umol/1, 87% of those predicted as not having CBD stones were correct. Patients with predicted mild attacks who have a high bilirubin on admission should therefore also be considered for ERC(P), although not necessarily urgently

ENDOSCOPIC SPHINCTEROTOMY AND STONE EXTRACTION

Confirmation of CBD stones at ERC(P) must lead to an immediate endoscopic sphincterotomy and active stone extraction.(29-33,60,69-71) The results shown in Table 1 are impressive in comparison to the results of treating acute gallstone pancreatitis in other British series. (14,15,54,67,72-76) It is perhaps worth recalling that a Hunterian lecture delivered on acute pancreatitis in 1966 revealed a mortality of biliary pancreatitis of 23%.(77) Undoubtedly, there has been a steady trend in the improved non-surgical management of these patients with a fall in mortality reported by most specialist centres. That the impact of urgent ERCP and ES in reducing morbidity is real, however, can only be substantiated by prospective randomized trials. The results of a recent trial(57) would indicate this to be so: morbidity was reduced from 54% (conventional treatment) to 18% (ERCP ±ES) and mortality was reduced from 18% to 2% respectively. Table 2 shows the collected results of ES from eight different series reported in the last 10 years, and illustrates the excellent trend in outcome by this form of treatment.

As can be seen from Table 1, patients will succumb to acute pancreatitis, even though they have had ERCP. This is because some patients have developed severe pancreatitis, even though they have passed all gallstones from the CBD. Eugene Opie, associate professor in pathology in the Johns Hopkins University, was well aware of this phenomenon: "The temporary lodgement of a calculus within the diverticulum (of Vater) may produce an extensive pancreatic lesion, and be finally expelled into the duodenum, the stone may be no longer demonstrable either at operation or at autopsy. Hence in a considerable number of cases the gallbladder will be found to be filled with gallstones, even though the bile ducts are free".(78)

The role of ERCP/ES is not just in the first 48-72 hours. Some patients will present at a later time, or deteriorate after showing initial improvement.

Series	Number	Complications due to ES	Deaths
Classen et al. 1978(29)	17	0	0
Van der Spuy 1981(30)	10	1	0
Kautz et al. 1982(33)	21	1	1
Reiman & Lux 1984(69)	15	0	0
Rosseland & Solhaug 1984(70)	29*	2	1
Neoptolemos et al. 1988(60)	37	3 (12**)	0
Safrany 1988(+)	158	15	5
Farkas et al. 1988‡(71)	284	15	5
Total		37 (6.5%)	12 (2.1%)

TABLE 2 Endoscopic sphincterotomy in acute gallstone pancreatitis in eight different series.

Referrals to units specialising in the management of these patients are likely to increase. Treatment in severe unremitting or deteriorating cases may include operative necrosectomy, drainage of abcesses, etc. and will be instituted beyond the initial 72 hour period. Where gallstones are the underlying pathology, laparotomy should be preceeded by ERCP ± ES, as CBD stones will often still be present. This avoids the need to explore the CBD, which can be extremely hazardous given the extent of peri-pancreatic necrosis, particularly around the CBD and duodenum.(66) Cholecystectomy may not always be necessary after an endoscopic sphincterotomy, because a wide sphincterotomy, will prevent further attacks.(79) This experience now includes over 50 such cases.

PATHOGENETIC ROLE OF PERSISTING COMMON BILE DUCT STONES

The hypotheses of the common channel, (4) migrating gallstones(17) and duodeno-pancreatic duct reflux(81-83) should not be perceived as mutully exclusive, but rather as each potentially important in initiating the attack of acute pancreatitis. Armstrong et al.(67) have identified some of the anatomi-

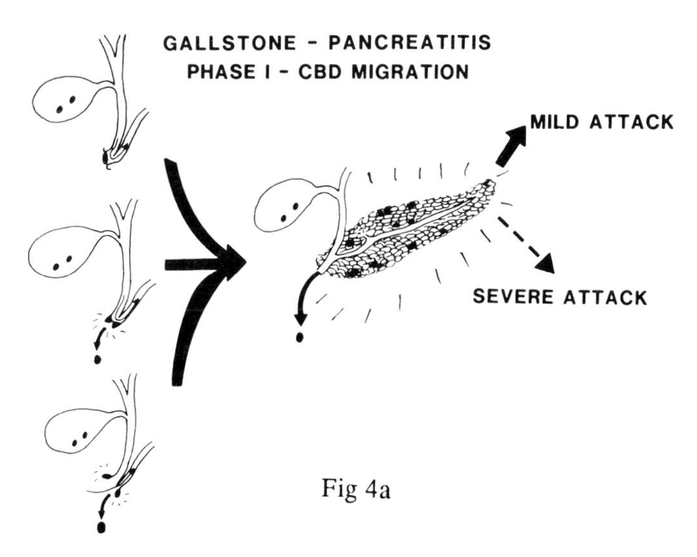

Fig 4a

Fig. 4 In Phase I, small "migrating" stones from the common bile duct (CBD) initiate the accack by any one of three mechanisms: duodeno-pancreatic reflux being the least likely. The outcome is usually a mild attack (Fig. 4a). In Phase " 11persisting" stones in the CBD block the secretion of pancreatic juice which now contains activated enzymes resulting in increased periductular inflammation with a tendency to severe (necrotizing) pancreatitis. The relative obstruction to the lower CBD results in an increased incidence of ascending cholangitis

cal factors which may predispose to bile reflux into the PD. Foulis has shown that gallstone pancreatitis is predominatly associated with periductular inflammation and necrosis.(84)

It is proposed that the process leading to severe gallstone pancreatitis has two phases (Fig.4). The attack of acute pancreatitis is initiated first by a process (phase I), involving the presence of activated enzymes within the pancreatic duct. This attack is usually mild as, if free drainage of the PD continues, inflammation of the pancreatic parenchyma will be limited. The patho-biochemical link between stones and the initiation of the attack remains speculative.(83,85) A severe attack supervenes if persisting CBD stones block the free drainage of activated enzymes from the PD (Phase II). Persisting CBD stones may block the PD duct if (i) they are large and permanently impact at the ampulla of Vater, or repeatedly impact and disimpact from the ampulla back into the CBD, or if (ii) they are small and numerous, and repeatedly traumatise the ampulla of Vater as they migrate into the duode-

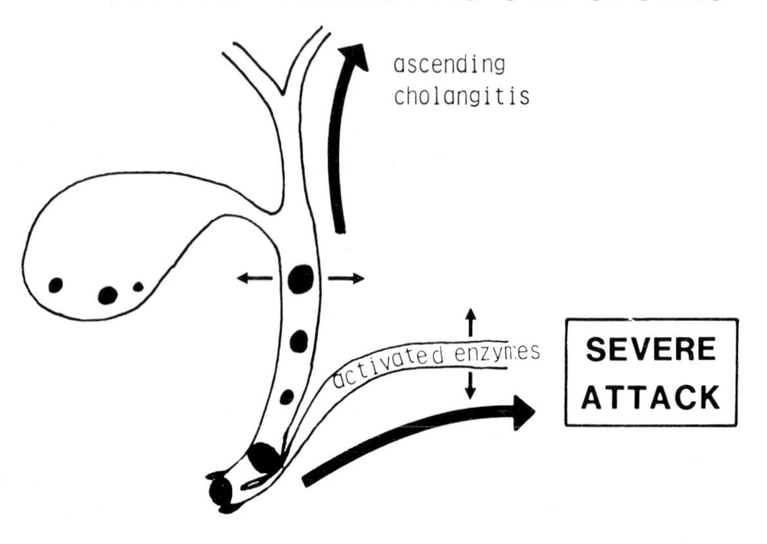

fig 4b

num causing marked ampullary oedema. The time scale between Phases I and II may be several hours or several days.

PATHOGENETIC ROLE OF DUODENAL PANCREATIC REFLUX

There has been some recent support (18,82,83,85) for this long expressed theory(80), but with little new substantive evidence. Although it is theoretically possible that reflux occurs as an initiating event, the proponents of reflux assume falsely that persisting CBD stones have no role in the progression of the attack. (82,83,85) There is, moreover, good evidence to refute use of the reflux theory to explain the initiation of acute gallstone pancreatitis.

One of the main premisses is that enterokinase and bacterial amidases are derived from duodenal reflux: (82,83,85) Both these potential pancreatic enzyme activating agents may well be present in bile, (86-88) but it is now clearly established that transduodenal sphincteroplasty or endoscopic sphincterotomy cause duodeno-choledochal reflux but not duodeno pancreatic duct reflux.(89)

Endosocopic sphinterotomy abolishes recurrent attacks of gallstone pancreatitis in patients with gallbladders in situ.(79) Gallstone pancreatitis is also extremely rare in patients who have had an ES for other reasons, of which more than 50,000 have now been performed world-wide.(90) McCutcheon, a great proponent of the duodenal reflux theory, wrote in 1964 "If the theory of duodenal reflux is correct, there are important implications for treatment ... sphincterotomy is contraindicated".(91) Quod erat demonstrandum!

THE ROLE OF SURGERY

Cholcystectomy has a well defined role in preventing further attacks of acute pancreatitis in patients with gallstones.

Opie recognised the importance of gallbladder stones following an attack. He described a 41 year old woman who had sustained recurrent attacks of acute pancreatitis and cautioned " ... acute haemorrhagic pancreatitis and consequent fat necrosis was doubtless caused by the passage of a small calculus similar to those so numerous in the gallbladder ... The clinical history makes it probable that similar calculi had been repeatedly expelled previous to the attack for which operation was performed but impaction in the diverticulum of Vater failed to occur. Removal of those still present in the gallbladder offered the best assurance of immunity from subsequent attacks".(78)

The optimum timing appears to be immediately following resolution of the attack and during the same admission.(15,25-28,92) Delaying cholectstectomy can result in recurrent attacks in 20% to 40% of cases.(15,25,26,92,93)

Ultrasound will determine the presence of gallstones in around 80% of cases if undertaken towards the end of an attack.(39) The detection rate can be improved using other techieques, including endoscopic duodenal collection of gallbladder bile following i.v. cholecystokinin-pancreazymin(94) and ERCP.(54)

Surgery has two other well defined roles in acute pancreatitis of all causes: internal drainage of large pseudocysts(95), and debridement and drainage of pancreatic abscesses.(96,97)

Although there is a generally accepted belief that removal of necrotic pancreatic material is beneficial, the surgical technique and timing remain unresolved. One school of thought which is gaining increasing acceptance is that surgery should be delayed until the second or third week.(98)

It may come as a surprise to some modern surgeons that this concept is not new. As early as 1903, Opie had written "During the primary collapse, little is to be gained by interference which would further impair the resistance of the patient; haemorrhage is rarely profuse and bears little relation to the severity of the condition. Should the individual survive the early symptoms of shock, infection of the gangrenous tissue and abscess formation limited to the lesser peritoneal cavity soon demand exploration and drainage. Septic fever, leucocytosis, and the presence of a palpable mass in the epigastrium indicate the necissity for operative interference".(78)

Delaying surgery for at least a week allows for relatively easy debridement of necrotic material by blunt dissection. This probably needs to be combined with an additional form of treatment, such as lavage into the pancreatic bed(98) or open packing via laparotostomy.(99)

Pancreatic surgery within the first few days of an attack will require a formal pancreatic resection.(100) Some studies have rejected this approach because of the high mortality, (100-102) but this may relate to its indiscriminate use in"severe" cases. There are cases in which the disease is so severe from the outset that death is inevitable within the first few days despite supportive measures. My own view is that such patients (provided that they are relatively young) ought to be treated by distal pancreatectomy, even though this view is difficult to justify completely by published date. Part of the problem lies in that such patients succumb so early that they never reach tertiary referral centres which have published the largest series on necrotizing pancreatitis.

The detection and quantitative assessment of pancreatic necrosis may now be achieved by high resolution contract-enhanced CT scanning techniques.(103-104) Estimation of the degree of pancreatic necrosis at open laparotomy is almost certainly unreliable.(105) Contrast enhanced CT when combined with adverse parameters such as a persistent high white cell count, C-reactive protein and, most of all, clinical judgement, may enable timely intervention for pancreatic debridement.(106) Professor Beger from Ulm, West Germany, has reported an impressively low mortality of 8% in this group of patients with such an approach.(98)

Whilst the arguments are persuasive, and are strengthened by the internal consistency of published date, there are relative weaknesses. There is little information on the natural history of pancreatic necrosis as determined by contrast enhanced CT, and no conclusive prospective randomised trial has compared operative with non-operative management. To what extent do areas of hypoperfusion of the pancreas merely reflect underperfusion of damaged, but otherwise recoverable, pancreatic tissue? To what extent does surgery interrupt the course of a patient who has pancreatic necrosis but who is otherwise showing signs of clinical improvement?

These reservations are perhaps overshadowed by the (re-discovered)-distinction between infected and non-infected pancreatic necrosis.(99,107,108) It appears that in the absence of surgical intervention, mortality from infected pancreatic necrosis approaches 100%, whereas in non-infected cases the mortality is around 10%.(107) Percutaneous sampling of pancreatic tissue during the attack now enables the presence of infection to be made reliably without resorting to surgery.(108,109)

This evidence suggests that intervention in patients with infected pancreatic necrosis is mandatory, and supports the routine use of antibiotics in patients with severe attacks, irrespective of aetiology. Evidence that antibiotics reduce the incidence of infection or that they improve outcome, however, is lacking. An additional reason for using antibiotics in severe gallstone pancreatitis is that there is an increased incidence of co-existing acute cholangitis.(60,61)

CONCLUSIONS

The development of prognostic criteria of severity and the introduction of new technology in the form of ERCP, contrast enhanced CT and interventional radiology, has considerably increased our understanding of the relationship between gallstones and pancreatitis and the evolution of necrotizing pancreatitis. Further application of these techniques will resolve some of the outstanding questions.

Paradoxically, our ability to treat acute pancreatitis is currently confined by the inherent limits of these new technologies. Clearly, additional approaches are required and the use of high dose fresh frozen plasma, for example, has produced some encouraging results.(110) Further progress will ultimately depend upon the elucidation of the biochemical relationship between acute pancreatitis and its systemic effects.

ACKNOWLEDGEMENTS

The art work and secretarial assistance of Mrs. Dilys Thomas and the support of the Department of Medical Photography, Dudley Road Hospital is gratefully acknowledged. I am indebted to many colleagues who collaborated in various studies reported here, and in particular to David Carr-Locke who undertood the great majority of ERCPs. Parts of this chapter formed the basis of a Hunterian Lecture delivered at the Royal College of Surgeons of England, Lincoln's Inn Fields, London, on 18th March 1988, and are reproduced with permission of the Editor of the Annals of the Royal College of Surgeons of England.

References

1. Johnson R. (Trans). The works of the famous chirurgeon Ambrose Pary. London, Mary Clark, 1678:565.
2. Fitz R. Acute pancreatitis. *Boston Med Surg J* 1889; *120:*181-229.
3. Opie EL. The relation of cholelithiasis to disease of the pancreas and to fat necrosis. *AM J Med Sci* 1901; *121*:27-43.
4. Opie EL. The etiology of acute haemorrhagic pancreatitis. *Johns Hopkins Hosp. Bull* 1901; *121*:182-8.
5. Bernard C. Lecors de physiologie experimental. Paris, J.B. Balliere, 1856.
6. Lancereaux E. Traite des maladies du foie et du pancreas. Paris, O. Poin 1899.
7. Moynihan B. Acute pancreatitis. *Ann Surg* 1925; *81*: 132-42.
8. Mayo WJ. The surgical treatment of pancreatitis. *Surg Gynecol Obstet* 1908; *6*:607-13.
9. Deaver JB, Sweet JE. Prepancreatic and peripancreatic disease. *J Am Med Ass* 1921; *77:* 194-7.
10. Mikkelsen O. Pancreatitis acuta; schwere falle, besonders hirischtligh ihrer konservativen Behandlung. *Acta Chir Scand* 1934; *75*: 373-415.
11. Glenn FG, Frey CF. Re-evaluation of the treatment of pancreatitis associated with biliary tract disease. *Ann Surg* 1964; *160:*723-6.
12. Frey CF. The operative treatment of pancreatitis. *Arch Surg* 1969; *98* : 406-17.
13. Ranson JH, Rifkind KM, Roses DF, Fink SD, Eng K, Spencer FC. Prognostic signs and the role of operative management in acute pancreatitis. *Surg Gynecol Obstet* 1974; *139:*69-81.
14. Imrie CW, Benjamin IS, Ferguson JC, *et al.* A single centre double-blind trial of Trasylol therapy in primary acute pancreatitis. *Br J Surg* 1978; *65:*337-41.
15. Osborne DH, Imrie CW, Carter DC. Biliary surgery in the same admission for gallstone-associated acute pancreatitis. *Br J Surg* 1981; *68:*758-61.
16. Blamey SL, Imrie CW, O'Neill J, Gilmour WH, Carter DC. Prognostic factors in acute pancreatitis. *Gut* 1984; *25*:1340-6.
17. Acosta JM, Ledesma CL. Gallstone migration as a cause of acute pancreatitis. *N Engl J Med* 1974;*290:*484-7
18. Cuschieri A, Cumming JGR, Wood RAB, Baker PR. Evidence for sphincter dysfunction in patients with gallstone associated pancreatitis: effect of ceruletide in patients undergoing cholecystectomy for gallbladder disease and gallstone associated pancreatitis. *Br J Surg* 1983; *71*:885-8.
19. Kelly TR. Gallstone pancreatitis: pathophysiology. *Surgery* 1976; *80*: No. 4:488-492
20. Mayer AD, McMahon MJ. Gallstones and acute pancreatitis - is the association underestimated? (Abstract). *Br J Surg* 1986; 71:905.
21. Acosta JM, Rossi R, Galli OMR, Pellegrini LA, Skinner DB. Early surgery for acute gallstone pancreatitis: Evaluation of a systematic approach. *Surgery* 1978; 83:367-70.

22. Stone HH, Fabian TC, Dunlop WE. Gallstone pancreatitis: biliary tract pathology in relation to time of operation. *Ann Surg* 1981; 194:305-10.
23. Mercer LC, Saltzstein EC, Peacock JB, Dougherty SH. Early surgery for biliary pancreatitis. *Am J Surg* 1984; 148:749-51.
24. Skinner DB. Should early surgical intervention be routinely recommended in the management of gallstone pancreatitis? Affirmative. In: Gitnick G. (ed).*Controversies in Gastroenterology*. London:Churchill Livingstone:1984: 197-203.
25. Paloyan D, Simonowitz D, Skinner DB. The timing of biliary tract operations in patients with pancreatitis associated with gallstones. *Surg Gynecol Obstet* 1975;141:737-739.
26. Ranson JHC. The timing of biliary surgery in acute pancreatitis. Ann Surg 1979; 189:654-62.
27. Kelly TR. Gallstone pancreatitis: The timing of surgery. *Surgery* 1980; 88:345-9.
28. Tondelli P. Stutz K, Harder F, Schuppisser JP, Allgower M. Acute gallstone pancreatitis: Best-timing for biliary surgery. *Br J Surg* 1982; 69:709-10.
29. Classen M. Ossenberg W. Wurbs D, Dammermann R, Hagenmuller F. Pancreatitis - an indication for endoscopic papillotomy? (Abstract). Endoscopy 1978; 10:223.
30. Van Spuy DS. Endoscopic sphincterotomy in the management of gallstone pancreatitis. *Endoscopy* 1981; 13:25-6.
31. Safrany L. Controversies in acute pancreatitis. In: Hollender LF (ed). Controversies in acute pancreatitis. New York:Springer-Verlag 1982:214-8.
32. Schott B, Neuhaus B, Portacarrero G, Krause S, Safrany L. Endoskopische papillotomie bei okuter bilaren pankreatitis. Klinikarzt 1982; 11:52-4.
33. Kautz G, Kohaus H, Keferstein R-D, Bunte H. Zur pathogenese und endoskopischen therapie der okuten bilaren pankreatitis. Klinikarzt 1982; 11:1202-12.
34. Gassendi P. Syntagma. Lyon, 1658. In: Harre R. (ed). *The philosophies of science. An introductory survey.* (2nd Edition). Oxford:Oxford University Press, 1985;88.
35. Lee HDP. (Trans). Plato, The Republic. Harmondsworth: Penguin Books Ltd. 1972.
36. Senn N. The surgery of the pancreas. Philadelphia: W.J. Dornan, 1886.
37. Dixon JA, Hillam JD. Surgical treatment of biliary tract disease associated with acute pancreatitis. *Am J Surg* 1970; 120:371-5.
38. Neoptolemos JP, Fossard DP, Berry JM. A prospective study of radionuclide biliary scanning in acute pancreatitis. *Ann Roy Coll Surg Engl* 1983; 65:180-2.
39. Neoptolemos JP, Hall AW, Finlay DF, Berry JM, Carr-Locke DL, Fossard DP. The urgent diagnosis of gallstones in acute pancreatitis: A prospective study of three methods. *Br J Surg* 1984; 71:230-3.
40. Van der Linden W, Kempi V, Edlund G. Function of liver, gallbladder and sphincter of Oddi after major surgery studied by computer-assisted cholescintigraphy and real-time ultrasonography. *Br J Surg* 1983; 70:497-501.

41. Weiner S, Gramatica L. Voegle LT, et al. Role of lymphatic system in pathogenesis of inflammatory disease in the biliary tract and pancreas. *Am J Surg* 1970; 119:55-61.
42. Fonseca C, Greenberg D, Rosenthall L, et al. 99m-Tc-IDA imaging in the differential diagnosis of acute cholecystitis and acute pancreatitis. *Radiology* 1979; 130:525-7.
43. Frank MS, Weissmann HS, Chun KJ, et al. Visualisation of the biliary tract with 99m-Tc-HIDA in acute pancreatitis. *Gastroenterology* 1980; 78:1167.
44. Glazer G. Murphy F, Clayden GS, et al. Radionuclide biliary scanning in acute pancreatitis. *Br J Surg* 1981; 68:766-70.
45. Serafini AN, Al-Sheikh W, Barkin JS, et al. Biliary scintigraphy in acute pancreatitis. *Radiology* 1982; 144:591-5.
46. Edlund G, Kempi V, Van der Linden W. Transient non-visualisation of the gallbladder by Tc-99m HIDA cholescintigraphy in acute pancreatitis: Concise communication. *J Nucl Med* 1982; 23:117-20.
47. Zeman RK, Segal HB, Caride V. Tc-99m HIDA cholescintigraphy in acute pancreatitis. Concise communication. *J Nucl Med* 1982; 23:117-20.
48. Ali A, Turner DA, Fordham EW. Tc-99m HIDA cholescintigraphhy in acute pancreatisis. Concise communication. *J Nucl Med* 1982; 23:867-9.
49. Blamey SL, Ballantyne KC, McArdle CS. A prospective study of radionuclide biliary scanning in acute pancreatitis. (Letter). *Ann Roy Coll Surg Engl* 1983; 65:352.
50. Frey CF. A strategy for the surgical management of gallstone pancreatitis. In : Beger HG, Buchler M (eds). *Acute pancreatitis.* Berlin:Springer-Verlag 1987.
51. McKay AJ, Imrie CW, O'Neil J, Duncan JG. Is an early ultrasound scan of value in acute pancreatitis? *Br J Surg* 1982; 69:369-72.
52. Blamey SL, Osborne DH, Gilmour WH, O'Neill J, Carter DC, Imrie CW. The early identification of patients with gallstone pancreatitis using clinical and biochemical factors only. *Ann Surg* 1983; 198:574-8.
53. Van Gossum A, Seferian V, Rodzynek JJ, Wetiendorff P, Cremer M. Delcourt A. Early detection of biliary pancreatitis. *Dig Dis Sci* 1984; 29: No 2:97-101.
54. Goodman AJ, Neoptolemos JP, Carr-Locke DL, Finlay DBL, Fossard DP. Detection of gallstones after acute pancreatitis. *Gut* 1985; 26:125-32.
55. Mayer AD, McMahon MJ. Biochemical identification of patients with gallstones associated with acute pancreatitis on the day of admission to hospital. *Ann Surg* 1985; 201:No. 1:68-75.
56. Davidson BR, Neoptolemos JP, Leese T, Carr-Locke DL. Biochemical prediction of gallstones in acute pancreatitis: a prospective study of three systems. *Br J Surg* 1988; 75:213-5.
57. Neoptolemos JP, Carr-Locke DL, London NJ, Bailey IA, James D., Fossard DP. Results of a controlled trial of urgent ERCP and endoscopic sphincterotomy in patients with acute pancreatitis due to gallstones. *Lancet* 1988; ii:979-83.

58. Matolo NM, Stadalnik RC, McGahan JP. Comparison of ultrasonography, computerised tomography and radio-nuclide imaging in the diagnosis of acute and chronic cholecystitis. *Am J Surg* 1982; 144:676-81.
59. London ND, Neoptolemos JP, Lavelle J, Bailey I, James R. Serial CT scanning in acute pancreatitis. *Br J Surg* 1989; 76 (in press).
60. Neoptolemos JP, Carr-Locke DL, London N, Bailey I, Fossard DP. ERCP findings and the role of endoscopic sphincterotomy in acute gallstone pancreatitis. *Br J Surg* 1988; 75:954-60.
61. Neoptolemos JP, Carr-Locke DL, Leese T, James D. Acute cholangitis in association with acute pancreatitis: incidence, clinical features and outcome in relation to ERCP and endoscopic sphincterotomy. *Br J Surg* 1987; 74: 1103-6.
62. McFadzean AJS, Yeung RTT. Acute pancreatitis due to Clonoarchis sinensis. *Trans R Soc Trop Med Hyg* 1966; 60:466-70.
63. Andrew DJ, Johnson SE. Acute suppurative cholangitis, a medical and surgical emergency. *Am J Gastroenterol* 1970; 54:141-54.
64. Ong GB, Adiseshiah M, Leong CH. Acute pancreatitis associated with recurrent pyogenic cholangitis. *Br J Surg* 1971; 58:891-4.
65. Ong GB, Lakn KH, Lam SK, Lim TK, Wong J. Acute pancreatitis in Hong Kong. *Br J Surg* 1979; 66:398-403.
66. Neoptolemos JP, Carr-Locke DL. ERCP in acute cholangitis and pancreatitis. In: *ERCP: Techniques and therapeutic applications.* New York:Elsevier Publishing Co. Inc. 1989 (in press).
67. Armstrong CP, Taylor TV, Jeacock J, Lucas S. The biliary tract in patients with acute gallstone pancreatitis. *Br J Surg* 1985; 72:551-5.
68. Neoptolemos JP, London N, Bailey I, Shaw D, Carr-Locke DL, Fossard DP, Moossa AR. The role of clinical and biochemical criteria and endoscopic retrograde cholangiopancreatography in the urgent diagnosis of common bile duct stones in acute pancreatitis. *Surgery* 1987; 100:732-42.
69. Riemann Von JF, Lux G. Therapeutische strategie bei der akuten pancreatitis (I). *Fortschr Med* 1984; 102:179-82.
70. Rosseland AR, Solhaug JH. Early or delayed endoscopic papillotomy (EPT) in gallstone pancreatitis. *Ann Surg* 1984; 199:165-7.
71. Farkas IE, Tulassay Z, Papp J. Endoscopic sphinterotomy in acute biliary pancreatitis: results of an international study. (Abstract). *Digestion* 1988: 40:80.
72. MRC Multicenter Trial. Death from acute pancreatitis. Lancet 1977; 2:632-5.
73. De Bolla AR, Obeid ML. Mortality in acute pancreatitis. *Ann Roy Coll Surg Engl* 1984; 66: 184-6.
74. Mayer AD, McMahon MJ, Benson EA, Axon ATR. Operations upon the biliary tract in patients with acute pancreatitis: aims, indications and timing. *Ann Roy Coll Surg Engl* 1984; 66:179-83.
75. Mayer AD, McMahon MJ, Corfield AP, Cooper MJ, Williamson RCN, Dickson AP, Shearer MG, Imrie CW. Controlled clinical trial of peritoneal lavage for the treatment of severe acute pancreatitis. *N Engl J Med* 1985; 312: 399-404.

76. Thomson HJ. Acute pancreatitis in North and North-East Scotland. *J Roy Coll Surg Edin* 1985; 30:104-11.
77. Trapnell JE. The natural history and prognosis of acute pancreatitis. *Ann Roy Coll Surg Engl* 1966; 38:265-87.
78. Opie EL. Disease of the pancreas. Its cause and nature. Philadelphia: JB Lippincott Company, 1903.
79. Davidson BR, Neoptolemos JP, Carr-Locke DL. Endoscopic sphincterotomy for common bile duct calculi in patients with gallbladder in situ considered unfit for surgery. *Gut* 1988; 29:114-20.
80. McCutcheon AD. Aetiological factors in pancreatitis. *Lancet* 1962; i:710-2.
81. McCutcheon AD. A fresh approach to the pathogenesis of pancreatitis.*Gut* 1968; 9:296-310.
82. Leading Article. Obstruction or reflux in gallstone-associated acute pancreatitis? *Lancet* 1988; i:95-7.
83. Barry RE. The pathogenesis of acute pancreatitis. (Leading Article). *Br Med J* 1988; 296:589
84. Foulis AK. Histological evidence of initiating factors in acute necrotising pancreatitis in man. *J Clin Path* 1980; 33:1125-31.
85. Keynes WM. The mythology of acute pancreatitis. *Infect Surg* 1987; 6:354- 68.
86. Hermon-Taylor J, Heywood GC. A rational approach to the specific chemotherapy of pancreatitis. *Scand J Gastroenterology* 1985; 117 (Suppl): 39-46.
87. Archibald E. The experimental production of pancreatitis in animals as a result of the residtance of the common duct sphincter. *Surg Gynecol Obstet* 1919; 28:529-45.
88. Armstrong CP, Taylor TV. Bile, bacteria and pancreatitis. *Surg Res Comm* 1988; 2:323-31.
89. Baker AR, Neoptolemos JP, Leese T, James DC, Fossard DP. Longterm follow-up of patients with side-to-side choledochoduodenostomy and transduodenal sphincteroplasty. *Ann Roy Coll Surg Eng* 1987; 68:253-7.
90. Cotton PB. Endoscopic management of bile duct stones (apples and oranges). *Gut* 1984; 25:587-97.
91. McCutcheon AD. Reflux of duodenal contents in the pathogenesis of pancreatitis. *Gut* 1964; 5:260-5.
92. Elfstrom J. The timing of cholecystectomy in patients with gallstone pancreatitis. *Acta Chir Scand* 1978; 144:487-90.
93. Kelly TR. Gallstone pancreatitis. *Arch Surg* 1974; 109:294-7.
94. Neoptolemos JP, Davidson BR, Winder AF, Vallance D. The role of duodenal bile crystal analysis in the investigation of "idiopathic" pancreatitis. *Br J Surg* 1988; 75:450-3.
95. Bradley EL III, Gonzalex AC, Clements JL. Acute pancreatic pseudocysts: incidence and implications. *Ann Surg* 1976; 184:734-7.
96. Warsaw AL, Jin G. Improved survival in 45 patients with pancreatic abscess. *Ann Surg* 1985; 202:408-17.

97. Bradley EL, Fulenwider JT. Open treatment of pancreatic abscess. *Surg Gynecol Obstet* 1984; 159:509-13.
98. Beger HG, Buchler M, Bittner R, Dettinger W, Block S, Nevalainen T. Necrosectomy and postoperative local lavage in patients with necrotizing pancreatitis: results of a prospective clinical trial. *World J Surg* 1988; 12:255-62.
99. Bradley EL, III. Management of infected pancreatic necrosis by open drainage. *Ann Surg* 1987; 206:542-50.
100. Kivilaakso E, Lempinen M, Makelainen A, Nikki P, Schroder T. Pancreatic resection versus peritoneal lavation for acute fulminant pancreatitis. *Ann Surg* 1984; 199:426-31.
101. Alexandre JH, Bohillot JL, Dhote J. Indications, techniques and results of resection of the pancreas. In: Berger HG, Buchler M (eds). Acute Pancreatitis. Berlin: Springer-Verlag 1987; 328-34.
102. Smadja C, Bismuth H. Pancreatic debridement in acute necrotizing pancreatitis: An obsolete procedure? *Br J Surg* 1986; 73:408-10.
103. Kivisaari L, Somer K, Standertskjold-Nordenstam C-G, Scaroder T, Kivilaakso E, Lempinen M. A new method for the diagnosis of acute haemorrhagic/necrotizing pancreatitis using contrast enhanced CT. *Gastrointest Radiol* 1984; 9:27-30.
104. Block S,. Maier W, Bittner R, Buchler M. Malfertheiner P, Beger HG. Identification of pancreatic necrosis in severe acute pancreatitis: imaging procedure versus clinical staging. *Gut* 1986; 27:1035-42.
105. Nordback I, Pessi T, Auvinen O, Aumo V. Determination of necrosis in necrotizing pancreatitis. *Br J Surg* 1985; 72:225-7.
106. Buchler M, Malfertheiner P, Shoetensack C, Uhl W, Beger HG. Sensitivity of antiproteases, complement factors and C-reactive protein in detecting pancreatic necrosis. Results of a prospective clinical study. *Int J Pancreatology* 1986; 1:227-35.
107. Beger HG, Block S, Bittner R. The significance of bacterial infection in acute pancreatitis. In: Beger HG, Buchler M (eds). *Acute Pancreatitis.* Berlin: Springer-Verlag 1987:79-86.
108. Van Sonnenberg E, Wittich GR, Casola G, Stauffer AE, Polansky AD, Coons HG, Cabrera OA, Gerver PS. Complicated pancreatic inflammatory disease: diagnostirc and therapeutic role of international radiology. *Radiology* 1985; 155:335-40.
109. Gerzof SG, Banks PA, Robbins AH, Johnson WC, Spechler J, Wetzner SM, Snider JM, Langevin RE, Jay ME. Early diagnosis of pancreatic infection by computed tomography-guided aspiration. *Gastroenterology* 1987; 93: 1315-20.
110. Leese T, Holiday M, Watkins M, Neoptolemos JP, Thomas WM. Preliminary results of a multicentre controlled clinical trial of high-volume fresh-frozen plasma therapy in prognostically severe acute pancreatitis. *Digestion* 1988; 40:97.

DISCUSSION

Hatfield: I agree wholeheartedly with the Leicester experience and message. The use of endoscopic sphincterotomy and gallstone removal is an important part of the management of the acutely ill patient with gallstone pancreatitis.

Imrie: I would like to sound a note of caution here. Sphincterotomies need to be performed by experts in centres with the necessary Intensive Care facilities and the resident staff to match. I fear an increased mortality rate from this disease if intervention by endoscopy is attempted by inexperienced people. Only 5 years ago this was one of the major contraindications for the use of diagnostic ERCP, let alone therapeutic ERCP, but now following this one study there is a general recommendation for not only diagnostic ERCP but therapeutic ERCP.

Jones: There is a danger of underestimating the competence of most District General Hospital Gastroenterologists who, by and large, are highly trained in endoscopic interventional procedures. From our experience in the South East, I would believe that the majority of District General Hospitals in the United Kingdom have gastroenterologists who can achieve 95% cannulations rates and an adequate and safe endoscopic sphincterotomy. Surely the majority of General Hospitals now have adequate Intensive Care Unit facilities to support this kind of service.

Russell: There are certainly centres with competent doctors but some do not have adequate endoscopes. Although one is training people, the facilities do not necessarily match and I think that one must not be complacent about this.

Trapnell: I am delighted that able endoscopists can be found in some district general hospitals, but I know that is not the case in all.

Hatfield: I support Mr Imrie's criticism. An ability to perform a technique does not mean that it can be performed equally well and safely in every single patient. Studies have shown clearly that the complication and success rate depends on the experience of the endoscopist. If one is tackling

2,000 ERCP's a year, one is going to be more able to manage difficult cases than if you only sees 50 cases a year. These factors all have to be considered when recommending complicated techniques. The other important factor is that a physician must not start an ERCP in this sort of patient unless he is prepared to go on and perform a therapeutic manouvre, if necessary. He must discuss it with the referring surgeon to start with, because a policy has to have been agreed before the endoscopy is performed.

Trapnell: The surgeon must be in town. This point has to emphasised.

Hatfield: Of course not all patients will need surgery if a stone cannot be cleared, instead one can drain that duct endoscopically and there are many ways to achieve this.

Trapnell: But if you cannot effect a clearance and a drainage, my own feeling would be that that patient should go to surgery.

Russell: No, most hospitals can now perform PTC's very competently. Once established, the catheter can be left in to drain.

Trapnell: A PTC in a dilated duct system can be achieved at low morbidity but a PTC in a non dilated system would carry a higher risk.

Imrie: Such an approach will only tackle the cholangitis, and will have no effect on the lower end of the duct if a stone remains.

Jones: That depends on the pathogenesis of pancreatitis with ductal stones. If, as I believe, a rise in pressure is important when a stone becomes impacted, then any form of decompression ought to be therapeutic.

Imrie: How can decompressing the biliary system help the pancreas?

Jones: I believe the existence of a common channel to have been proven. Elegant radiological and polyvinyl cast studies have shown that a communication exists between the system in at least 85% of people.

McMahon: The best animal model of gallstone related pancreatitis is probably the opossum. This creature has a common channel, with a sphincter around it, independent bile and pancreatic ducts, and a gall bladder and cystic duct. Senninger and Moody et al (1) showed that if the pancreatic duct is ligated, oedematous pancreatitis results. If the common channel is ligated, haemorragic pancreatitis develops. If the pancreatic duct and the bile duct above the junction of the two are ligated independently, so that there is no cross communication between them, haemorragic pancreatitis results - suggesting that a component and perhaps a determinant of the severity of gallstone pancreatitis is concomitant obstruction of the bile duct. It may be important to decompress the bile duct and it may help the pancreas, we do not know. The only study I know of which has looked at the common channel theory and the incidence of reflux into the pancreatic duct during the acute stage of pancreatitis, was a study by Acosta, in 1988.(2) Operative cholangiograms were taken and reflux was present in less than a quarter of the patients(23%), so it is difficult to argue that the common channel theory is an 80% phenomenon.

Neoptolemos: I accept that, but Acosta also demonstrated that tiny stones which are being passed can cause oedema, and that once you accept that oedema may be sufficient to cause pancreatic duct reflux then one does not need the rigid arithmetical restrictions that those investigating it anatomically have said is necessary. Remember also that it may not be possible to show reflux in patients with established pancreatitis by operative colangiograms. In the Leicester study the incidence of pancreatograms was significantly lower in patients with common bile duct stones; this was curious and remains unexplained.

Salmon: I was interested by the data from the 19 centre European study on urgent sphincterotomy, showing a complication rate of 5%. This figure is almost exactly the same as our own at the Middlesex for over a thousand sphincterotomies, so there does not seem to be an increased risk.

Neoptolemos: A number of the enthusiasts are reporting complications relating to the procedure, not to the overall outcome, which I think is the wrong way to do it.

The urgent application of ERCP will limit the necrosis to some extent. The whole aim is to try and dampen down the attack. The other indication is in the patient who is not getting better. There are different times and different situations for its use.

Trapnell: If a patient comes into the casualty with pancreatitis at 7 o'clock on a Tuesday evening, when does he or she receive their sphincterotomy?

Neoptolemos: At Dudley Road Hospital the patient would be fully assessed, started on antibiotics and would be placed on the first available ERCP list. That may or may not be within 72 hours but that is to do with the poor resources, which is a real problem.

Shorvon: Once the decision has been made that severe pancreatitis is the likely diagnosis and yet at endoscopy a stone is not seen on the radiograph, then a sphincterotomy should still be considered, because a stone may be there after all.

Neoptolemos : Yes, but it is important to remember that the mortality rate from endoscopic sphincterotomy in that sort of group is probably about 1 or 2%.

Shorvon: I am conservative and feel one should not be doing an ERCP except when one expects stones. I am then saying that having made that decision if they are not seen one should proceed to sphincterotomy anyway, after which the stones may unexpectedly appear.

Neoptolemos : I think that is dangerous. The mortality has been reduced to about 2% if sphincterotomy is done only in those with common bile duct stones. If you are going to start doing this in the group of patients without common bile duct stones, there is a risk of increasing the morbidity, not decreasing it.

Shorvon: I accept that there is a risk, but I have seen on several occasions stones which have been missed on ERCP films, particularly small stones, because optimum radiographs have not been available. In patients with severe pancreatitis conditions are often not optimum for good radiographic production and the stones are often small.

Hatfield: The issue is not easy. Certainly, occasionally following a sphincterotomy a stone is found when a balloon catheter is pulled down an apparently normal bile duct. On the other hand if a sphincterotomy was performed routinely, regardless of the presence of a calculus or not, the complication rate would rise. In certain circumstances I feel it is justified but not in all.

Trapnell: Dr Leese, can you update us on the fresh frozen plasma trial?

Leese: The results of the low volume trial are known (3). Fresh frozen plasma can be used to supplement serum alpha-2-macroglobulin levels. High volume fresh frozen plasma is now being studied to see if the alpha-2-macroglobulin levels can be elevated to within the normal range, and if a clinical benefit results. Fresh frozen plasma has no effect on acute phase protein levels because the quantity of these proteins in fresh frozen plasma is insignificant compared to the amount mobilised in the acute phase response.

Patients with prognostically severe acute pancreatitis are randomised into two groups. They receive either 24 units of fresh frozen plasma over 3 days, or human albumin solution, as control, which has the colloid effect without the potentially beneficial specific proteins. It is a multicentre trial and the Imrie prognostic criteria are being used to select prognostically severe patients, using a score of three or more. Unfortunately only 15% to 20% of patients are predicted severe on the Imrie score within six hours of diagnosis. Previous studies using the Glasgow criteria at 48 hour have reported that as many as 30% of patients with pancreatitis were predicted as severe. For our statistical analysis we need a minimum of 96 patients. The low sensitivity of the Imrie score within six hours of diagnosis has slowed recruitment of patients into the trial so that in the first year only 32 were entered instead of the estimated 45. In the group receiving fresh frozen plasma it has already been shown that alpha-2- macroglobulin levels can be maintained within the normal range. The trial must continue to see if any clinical benefit results. Of the 32 patients included so far, 15 were randomised to the control group, amongst whom we have had four deaths. Of the 17 patients in the treatment arm there has been only one death.

McMahon: I wish to encourage this study. Data which we have presented recently at the Surgical Research Society does sugggest that there is a problem with the anti- protease defence mechanism in severe pancreatitis and that there is a different complexing of trypsin to the anti-proteases than seen normally. The complexes formed with alpha-2-macroglobulin have a delayed clearance. I wonder whether it is not just a question of providing the alpha-2- macroglobulins but also enhancing clearing of the complexes which are formed, because they retain biological activity to smaller molecular weight substrates and they may play an important part in the pathogenesis of the systemic component of the attack.

Neoptolemos: Does this trial not illustrate a problem in running a biochemical experiment for acute pancreatitis? There are so many putative mechanisms being tackled, not only in the test arm with fresh frozen plasma incorporating for example fibronectin, but also by the albumin in the control arm: Phospholipase A2 is produced in pancreatitis, phosphilipase A2 will split off fatty acids from cell membranes and these are toxic. Albumin will counter this by carrying the fatty acids.

Larvin: It has been said that we do not have a treatment of proven value. It is argued that if any of the therapies evaluated over the past 20 years had been of great benefit then a clear advantage would have been shown consistently. Is this not a case of asking for the improbable, a "barn door effect"? Should we not accept simply that the recruitments of patients were inadequate? It may be that the disease is so complex that we have to combine different medical treatments and surgical strategies to produce a useful result.

Imrie: I would agree and I would go further and say that probably the different major aetiologies need to be considered separately. It may be that peritoneal lavage should be re-examined for those with an alcohol aetiology. I suspect there is a completely different peritoneal event in patients with alcohol-induced pancreatitis compared to the gallstone group.

Zentler- Munro: Dr Salmon was describing what amounts to a cascade phenomenon. Timing will matter considerably. To what extent have the drug trials considered that timing might be vital? By analogy with infarction and thrombolysis, one may be treating patients in vast numbers, only a minority of whom may actually need that treatment.

Neoptolemos: That is the fundamental fallacy of the specific drug approach aimed at switching the pancreas off. These patients are admitted with established acute pancreatitis. One must lessen the systemic effect and limit the damage to the pancreas in a mechanical or operative way. To believe the process of pancreatitis can be stopped with drugs is philosophically wrong.

Salmon : If one was able to get the patient at the appropriate time, knowing what was going to develop, an attempt to stop this cascade would be the right approach. The problem is that when the patients arrive all these things have happened.

Zentler-Munro: We are now talking about giving streptokinase to patients at home. Will the same come about for pancreatitis?

Imrie: I do not think so. I fear many general practitioners fail to consider the diagnosis of pancreatitis. If pancreatitis is the cause, the best action is to get the patient to hospital quickly where they can receive IV fluids, and improve the microcirculation of the pancreas. That may be the single most important therapeutic advance that can possibly occur with this disease, getting the GP to consider the diagnosis and start IV fluids early.

Keynes: Mr Neoptolemos, why do you think that a sphincterotomy remains patent for a long time?

Neoptolemos: Follow-up barium studies will demonstrate refluxing rapidly up the biliary tree without any difficulty; never into the pancreatic duct, because there is a separate pancreatic duct sphincter.

Imrie: If duodenal reflux was the cardinal, pivotal factor in developing acute pancreatitis, there are many patients who have had endoscopic sphincterotomies who you would expect to be relapsing. This is not the case.

References

1. Senninger N, Moody FG, Coelho JC, Van Buren DH. The role of biliary obstruction in the pathogenesis of acute pancreatitis in the opossum. *Surg* 1986; 99: 688-93.
2. Acosta JM, Pellegrini CA, Skinner DB. Aetiology and pathogenesis of acute biliary pancreatitis. *Surg* 1980; 88: 118-25.
3. Leese T et al. Multicentre clinical trial of low volume fresh frozen plasma therapy in acute pancreatitis. *Br J Surg* 1987; 74:907-911.

HOW DOES ALCOHOL DAMAGE THE PANCREAS

Mr M J McMahon
Consultant Surgeon
Leeds General Infirmary

Introduction

The association between alcohol and pancreatitis was first recognised by Fitz in 1889. It has become clear that people who drink alcohol run the risk of acute and chronic pancreatitis but relatively little is known about causative mechanisms. One might think that it would have been a more common problem in days gone by, according to the epidemiology of alcohol consumption in the United Kingdom, and it is curious that no lay term for acute and chronic pancreatitis has arisen. Recently, that is to say in the last forty years, there have been increases in the amount of alcohol consumed in the United Kingdom, and in the prevalence of both acute and chronic pancreatitis. The changing pattern of acute pancreatitis was first documented in Gothenberg. Gallstones were associated with the majority of attacks of acute pancreatitis in 1957, but more recently alcohol had become the major causative factor (1). A similar trend, though not as dramatic, is now being seen in this country.

In 1975 Trapnell recorded his experience of 64 cases of chronic pancreatitis (2), of which about half were due to alcohol. As with acute pancreatitis, there was a trend towards a progressively greater percentage of cases which could be attributed to excess consumption of alcohol.

In 1960 John Howard wrote " .... but the fact that alcoholic pancreatitis is a distinct entity with characteristics quite separate from those of gallstone pancreatitis; a natural history almost entirely different from other forms - this fact has not been fully appreciated. In Leeds attacks due to alcohol occur most frequently in young or middle aged men, many after attempting to drown themselves in cheap Mediteranean wine whilst on holiday abroad. Because of this the peak incidenceof acute pancreatitis related to alchol is during the summer months. Patients who develop acute pancreatitis due to gallstones are often elderly ladies who develop their pancreatitis in the autumn. Others have recorded this seasonal incidence, and dietary factors may play a part. There are suggestions that pancreatitis associated with gallstones is more severe then that due to alcohol. This has not been substantiated and may depend upon the manner in which the diagnosis is made.

Although there are some differences, there is broad similarity in the biochemical changes found in both types of acute pancreatitis. Plasma levels differ slightly, but not singnificantly (4), apart from amylase, which is often lower.(5) This difference has been appreciated for many years, and is thought to reflect the fact that the pancreas does not have the capacity to produce enzymes if it has been damage chronically by alcohol. Another reason may be that the factors which trigger an attack of alcoholic pancreatitis do not induce the back diffusion of enzymes to the extent which occurs in gallstone related attacks. The concentration of enzymes in peritoneal fluid is not greatly different in the two types of attack ,(6) but the role of peritoneal enzymes in the pathogenesis of the attack might be more important in patients with alcohol related pancreatitis. In the UK multicentre study of peritoneal lavage in severe pancreatitis there was no overall influence of treatment upon survival. (7) When results were analysed according to aetiology there was the suggestion that alcohol related patients did better when they were lavaged, but numbers were too small to be susceptible to statistical analysis (23 attacks due to alcohol). A randomised study of peritoneal lavage in patients with alcoholic pancreatitis was reported from Atlanta,(8) and showed a significant influence of the therapy.

Differences exist in the relationship between alcohol and acute and chronic pancreatitis. There is no doubt that an acute debauch with little past history of alcohol intake can result in acute pancreatitis, but chronic pancreatitis is more usually due to chronic alcohol intake. Ammann has shown that the pancreas is not necessarily irreversibly damaged by alcohol, even following relapsing acute attacks .(9)

MECHANISMS OF PANCREATITIS DUE TO ALCOHOL

There are various mechanisms by which alcohol is thought to damage the pancreas. These include an influence upon neural control of the pancreas, an influence upon the endocrine stimulation of secretion, damage to pancreatic cells by the toxic effects of ethanol, alterations in bile or pancreatic juice, and interference with ampullary function.

Darie, Ekholm and Edlund studied the effect of long-term alcohol ingestion upon the ultrastructure of the rat pancreas .(10) They demonstrated an accumulation of lipid droplets in the acinar cells, swelling of the mitochondria, and foci of cytoplasmic degeneration. When Reber et al carried out similar studies, however, they could not reproduce this damage nor could they demonstrate the progression to chronic pancreatitis which others had shown .(11) It was in 1986 that Heij and his colleagues pointed out that all the experimental studies that had shown pancreatic damage caused by alcohol ingestion were in male rats, whereas studies in female rats produced less pronounced morphological change. (12) This interesting observation may have a parallel in patients. Although drinking is now very common in young women and certainly leads to chronic pancreatitis, acute pancreatitis due to alcohol is almost confined to men.

Toxicity of ethanol upon the acinar cells

It is unclear if there is a linear relationship between alcohol consumption and pancreatic disease although some studies suggest that there is. (13) It is also unclear why 8-10 years of alcohol consumption is generally required before chronic pancreatitis becomes symptomatic, and why organ specificity and selectivity appears to exist with respect to alcohol damage.

It is unlikely that acetaldehyde, an end-product of the oxidative metabolism of ethanol which contributes to hepatic damage caused by alcohol, is responsible for the induction of acute or chronic pancreatitis, because the pancreas has limited ability to oxidise ethanol. Non-oxidative metabolism does occur in the pancreas, resulting in the formation of fatty acid ethyl esters. (14) These esters can act as a shuttle for fatty acid between cellular binding sites and mitochrondria, where they may be hydrolysed to release fatty acids, which have the power to uncouple oxidative phosphorylation. The normal method of secretion of secretory enzymes from the pancreas is by vacuole formation. Zymogen granules and lysozomes are produced in the endoplasmic reticulum and become concentrated in separate vacuoles. This process has been shown to change under certain circumstances such as super-secretion of the gland with a CCK analogue, and result in pancreatitis. Instead of separate lines of vacuole development both secretory and lysozomal enzymes may develop in a single vacuole, so that the secretory zymogens such as trypsinogen are activated by lysosomal enzymes such as cathepsin B. Alternatively, the two vacuoles can commence development separately, but because they are thin walled and abnormal, coelescence occurs (crinophagy) with resulting autoactivation of zymogen. This mechanism has been suggested in rats that were given oral ethanol by the finding of morphological changes similar to those of chronic pancreatitis coupled with the presence of cathepsin B in zymogen granules. (15) It has not been confirmed that it occurs in man. Evidence to support the direct toxic effect of ethanol includes the short history in some patients, and the changes in the histology which can be found in the pancreas of heavy drinkers who do not have clinical pancreatitis. Against it, apparently, is the delay which may be of several days in some patients between an acute "binge" and the presentation of acute pancreatitis. This has not been adequately explained. Also unclear is the fact that although some patients develop acute pancreatitis after an alcholic debauch, many do not.

Acute pancreatitis occurs in patients with familial hyperlipidaemia (Types I and V) in whom chylomicron levels are elevated, and Cameron has shown that chronic alcohol abusers with Type IV hyperlipidaemia (raised levels of lipoproteins) convert to Type V (chylomicronaemia) when challenged with a fatty meal, and may develop abdominal pain similar to acute pancreatitis, with elevation of amylase. (16,17) Thus in chronic alcohol abusers, an alcoholic debauch or a fatty meal can lead to elevated chylomicrons. Hydrolysis of triglycerides in and around the pancreas under the influence of pancreatic lipase could lead to local release of free fatty acids. These are toxic and may produce cell injury by releasing oxygen-derived free radicals such as 0_2 which can cause peroxidation of membrane lipids (18), thus liberating more pancreatic lipase and so facilitating an escalation of the process. It is difficult to accept that this mechanism plays a central role in the production of pancreatitis in patients who abuse alcohol because hyperlipidaemia is uncommon. In experimental animals Ramo showed that the severity of acute pancreatitis induced by the infusion of bile into the pancreatic duct was increased by a combination of chronic ethanol consumption and a fat-rich diet (19).

Ethanol and the composition of pancreatic juice

Alcohol has been shown to have a variety of effects upon the composition of pancreatic juice. For example, short term administration of alcohol intravenously or intrajejunally caused a reduction in pancreatic juice volume and in the concentrations of bicarbonate and enzymes (20), and pancreatic juice stimulated by injection of secretion and cholecystokinin (CCK) from chronic alcohol abusers (>100 g alcohol per day) was found to contain greater concentrations of protein than the juice from non-alcoholic control patients. (21) The relevance of these changes to the causation of pancreatitis remains unclear, but they may be important to the 'protein plug' hypothesis which has been developed by Sarles and his group. According to this hypothesis chronic pancreatitis is initiated by deposits of protein which block small ducts within the pancreas. (22) It is postulated that protein precipitates, which can aggregate into plugs, form as a result of the high concentration of protein within the pancreatic juice and a relative deficit of a protein of approximately 13500 D which normally acts to maintain other proteins in solution in the juice. This protein has been extracted from intraduct stones and protein plugs and termed Pancreatic Stone Protein. (23, 24)

Sarles did not consider activation of enzymes within the juice to be an important component of the formation of protein precipitates (24). Rinderknecht et al confirmed the finding of increased protein concentration in the stimulated pancreatic juice of chronic alcohol abusers, but also found changes in the proportions of the different types of trypsinogen, with a five-fold increase in anionic trypsinogen, and an increase in the ratio of trypsinogen to trypsin inhibitor. (25) They postulated that the distorted zymogen:inhibitor ratios could facilitate premature activation of pancreatic zymogens.

Influence of alcohol upon permeability of the pancreatic duct

Using an experimental preparation which utilises the perfused cat pancreas, Reber's group have shown that alcohol, administered orally caused increased permeability of the pancreatic duct. (26) In control animals the duct was permeable to molecules up to 3000 D, but after alcohol it became permeable to molecules up to 20,000 in size. Transductal migration of enzymes, bile etc. might result in peri-ductal inflammation and fibrosis. There is no evidence to support this mechanism in man.

Alcohol and the Spincter of Oddi

It has been suggested that alcohol causes pancreatic duct obstruction secondary to duodenitis (17), or by inducing spasm of the sphincter of Oddi .(28) Using endoscopic manometry, Viceconte showed that ethanol, given intragastrically or intravenously, caused a significant inhibition of Sphincter of Oddi pressure. (29) Okazaki et al used a microtransducer inserted through a duodenoscope to record pressures in the ampullary sphincter and in the pancreatic duct .(30) In patients with alcoholic chronic pancreatitis there was some degree of increase in basal sphincter pressure and a marked increase in pancreatic duct pressure compared to controls. It has also been suggested, but without foundation, that alcohol causes reflux of duodenal juice or bile into the pancreatic duct and thus permits activation of zymogens by enterokinase. (31)

Interference with the control of pancreatic secretion

Tiscornia and Dreiling suggest that alcohol produces a secretory influence upon the pancreas by inhibiting the normal down-regulation, inhibitory, or 'brake' reflexes which reduce pancreatic juice production as the stomach empties after a meal .(32) This results in increased cholinergic secretomotor activity and thus an enhanced sectetory response to secretin and

CCK. Whilst the evidence for this mechanism is derived from experimental animals indirect support for it in man comes from a randomised study of vagotomy and Billroth II gastrectomy in patients with recurrent acute pancreatitis caused by alcohol. (33) The operation reduced recurrent pancreatitis to 6% over a period of up to 26 months follow-up compared to 73% in patients managed conservatively. Further support for the importance of pancreatic secretory pressure as a cause of pain in chronic pancreatitis is provided by a randomised study of enzyme supplementation using granular pancreatin. (34) Pancreatin administration caused a significant reduction in pain - probably by reducing the CCK response to meals and hence lowering the secretory pressure within the gland. In this case the 'brake' mechanism would have been boosted by the intraduodenal presence of enzymes from the pancreas.

Conclusion

Many alternative mechanisms have been proposed to link alcohol consumption with acute and chronic pancreatitis. Which of these are important in man remains unknown, and it is possible that multiple factors are operative, involving not only alcohol but also food, other types of drink and tobacco. It is important that the relationship between alcohol and pancreatic diseases are understood more completely if the present upward trend in the prevalence of pancreatic disease is to be reversed.

References

1. Svensson J-O, Nordback B, Bokey EL, Edlund Y. Changing pattern in aetiology of pancreatitis in an urban Swedish area. *Br J Surg* 1979; 66: 159-161.
2. Trapnell JE. Chronic relapsing pancreatitis: a review of 64 cases. *Br J Surg* 1979; 66: 471.
3. Howard JM. In: Surgical Diseases of the Pancreas. Ed. JM Howard and GL Jordan. Pitman, London. 1960. pp 190.
4. Dubick MA, Mar G, Mayer AD, Majumdar APN, McMahon MJ, Geokas MC. Digestive enzymes and protease inhibitors in plasma from patients with acute pancreatitis. *Pancreas* 1987; 2: 187-194.
5. McMahon MJ, Mayer AD. Comparison of the clinical features of acute pancreatitis due to gallstones and alcohol. In: Pancreatitis - Concepts and Classification. Ed. KE Gyr, MV Singer, H Sarles. Elsevier Science Publishers, Amsterdam 1984; 170-388.
6. Dubick MA, Mayer AD, Majumdar APN, Mar G, McMahon MJ, Geokas MC. Biochemical studies in peritoneal fluid from patients with acute pancreatitis. Relationship to aetiology. *Dig Dis Sci* 1987; 32: 305-312.
7. Mayer AD, McMahon MJ, Corfield AP, et al. Controlled clinical trial of peritoneal lavage for the treatment of severe acute pancreatitis. *New Engl J* Med 1985; 399-404.
8. Stone HH, Fabian TC. Peritoneal dialysis in the treatment of acute alcoholic pancreatitis. *Surg Gynec Obstet* 1980; 150: 878-882.
9. Ammann RW, Buehler H, Bruehlmann W, Kehl O, Muench R, Stamm B. Acute (non progressive) alcoholic pancreatitis: prospective longitudinal study of 144 patients with recurrent alcoholic pancreatitis. *Pancreas* 1986; 1: 195-203.
10. Darle N, Ekholm R, Edlund Y. Ultrastructure of the rat exocrine pancreas after long-term intake of ethanol. *Gastroenterology* 1970; 58: 62-72.
11. Reber HA, Johnson FE, Montgomery CK, Carl WR, Wong MF. The affect of chronic alcohol ingeston on rat pancreas. *Gastroenterology* 1977; 72: 1117.
12. Heij HA, Obertop H, Westbroek DL, Tenkate FW. The effects of long term alcohol consumption on morphology and function of the exocrine pancreas of the rat. *Surgical Research Communications* 1987; 1 : 115-126.
13. Durbec JP, Sarles H. Multicentre survey of the aetiology of pancreatic diseases. Relationship between the relative risk of developing chronic pancreatitis and alcohol protein and lipid consumption. *Digestion* 1978; 18: 337-350.
14. Laposta EA, Lange LG. Presence of nonoxidative ethanol metabolism in human organs commonly damaged by ethanol abuse. *Science* 1986; 231 : 497-499.
15. Singh M. Alcoholic pancreatitis in rats fed ethanol in a nutritionally adequate liquid diet. *Int J Pancreatology* 1987; 2: 311-324.

16. Cameron JL, Capuzzi DM, Zuidema GD, Margolis S. Acute pancreatitis with hyperlipaemia: evidence for a persistent defect in lipid metabolism. *Am J Med* 1974; 56: 482.
17. Cameron JL, Zuidema GD, Margolis S. A pathogenesis for alcoholic pancreatitis. *Surgery* 1975; 77: 754.
18. Sanfey H, Bulkley GB, Cameron JL. The role of oxygen derived free radicals in the pathogenesis of acute pancreatitis. *Ann Surg* 1984; 200: 405-413.
19. Ramo OJ. Antecedent long-term ethanol consumption in combination with different diets alters the severity of experimental acute pancreatitis in rats.*Gut* 1987; 28: 84-89 .
20. Marin GA, Ward NL, Fischer R. Effects of ethanol on pancreatic and biliary secretions in humans. *Dig Dis* 1973; 18: 825-833.
21. Sahel J, Sarles H. Modifications of pure human pancreatic juice induced by chronic alcohol consumption. *Dig Dis Sci* 1979; 24: 897-905.
22. Nakamura K, Sarles H, Payan H. Three-dimensional reconstruction of the pancreatic ducts in chronic pancreatitis. *Gastroenterology* 1972; 62: 942-949.
23. De Caro A, Lohse J, Sarles H. Characterisation of a protein isolated from pancreatic calculi of men suffering from chronic calcifying pancreatitis. *Biochem Biophys Res Comm* 1979; 87: 1176-1182.
24. Guy O, Robles-Diaz G, Adrich Z, Sahel J, Sarles H. Protein content of precipitates present in pancreatic juice of alcoholic subjects and patients with chronic calcifying pancreatitis. *Gastroenterology* 1983; 84: 102-107.
25. Rinderknecht H, Stace NH, Renner IG. Effects of chronic alcohol abuse on exocrine pancreatic secretion in man. *Dig Dis Sci* 1985; 30: 65-71.
26. Wedgwood KR, Adler G, Kern H, Reber HA. Effects of oral agents on pancreatic duct permeability. A model of acute alcoholic pancreatitis. *Dig Dis Sci* 1986; 31: 1081-1088.
27. Herman RE, Davis JH. The role of incomplete pancreatic duct obstruction in the etiology of pancreatitis. *Surgery* 1960; 48: 318-329.
28. Pirola RC, Davis E. Effects of ethyl alcohol on sphincteric resistance at the choledocho-duodenal junction in man. *Gut* 1968; 9: 557-560.
29.Viceconte G. Effects of ethanol on the Sphincter of Oddi: an endoscopic manometric study. *Gut* 1983; 24: 20-27.
30. Okazaki K, Yamamoto Y, Kagiyama S, Tamura S, Sakamoto Y, Morita M, Yamamoto Y. Pressure of papillary sphincter zone and pancreatic main duct in patients with alcoholic and idiopathic chronic pancreatitis. *Int J Pancreatology* 1988; 3: 457-468.
31. Grant D. Acute necrotising pancreatitis - a role for enterokinase. *Int J Pancreatology* 1986; 1 : 167-183.
32. Tiscornia OM, Dreiling DA. Physiopathogenic hypothesis of alcoholic pancreatitis: Supranormal ecbolic stimulation of the 'pancreon units

secondary to the loss of the negative component of pancreas innervation. *Pancreas* 1987; 2: 604-612.
33. Stone HH, Mullins RJ, Scovill WA. Vagotomy plus Billroth II gastrectomy for the prevention of recurrent alcohol-induced pancreatitis. *Ann Surg* 1985; 201 : 684-689.
34. Isaksson G, Ihse I. Pain reduction by an oral pancreatic enzyme preparation in chronic pancreatitis. *Dig Dis Sci* 1983; 28: 97-102.

DISCUSSION

Neoptolemos: It is an interesting phenomenon that if alcohol is given to normal people and manometric studies are performed, the sphincter seems to relax. On the other hand if one performs the experiment on the opossum an opposite effect is seen, and the sphincter is more sensitive. What has not been done is a study of the effect of alcohol on the ampullary sphincter in patients who have had an attack of alcohol pancreatitis. They may respond in a different way to the normal population.

McMahon: This was done in 1988 by Okazaki and co-worker(30). A study was published where a microtransducer was placed in the terminal pancreatic duct and in the sphincter itself. The sphincter behaved relatively normally in patients with chronic pancreatitis, but pancreatic duct pressures were higher. This may have been ascribed to increased viscosity of the pancreatic juice. I agree that more investigation in acute pancreatitis is required.

Zentler-Munro: A lot of what you said made me think of cystic fibrosis, which is extraordinary because even in young patients where the pancreas has not atrophied, acute pancreatitis is not common. Yet these people have increased protein secretion in many biological fluids, the protein is abnormally structured and it behaves in an abnormal way, and there are other similarities. Another interesting fact comes from a study by Marks and Banks (1965) in which an increase in sweat sodium was seen in heavy drinkers who had pancreatitis, but not in those who had cirrhosis; not to the level diagnostic of C.F., but to an intermediary level of the order that is found in the presumed heterozygotes of the disease. One must consider whether there is a common aetiological link between the pancreatic damage in the two diseases.

McMahon: Despite the fact that there are changes in the juice, these may not be the trigger factors that are necessary for acute pancreatitis.

Imrie: The same group have looked recently at a group of patients who had a single attack of acute pancreatitis related to alcohol abuse, who were known to be heavy drinkers. A follow-up study involved both pancreatic function tests and ERCP in those who continued drinking and a small group who stopped. The pancreatic function deterioration and duct changes were arrested in those who stopped drinking, and in some patients there was even an improvement. All those who continued to drink suffered a deteriorating situation, both structurally and functionally.

McMahon: That differs a little from the work of Rudi Ammann who has suggested that although there is a correlation between deterioration and continued drinking, nevertheless some patients continued to drink but had no further pain and showed no deterioration in function.

Imrie: I am not sure how closely controlled Ammann's patients were. There are vast numbers. Ammann has contentiously documented a regression and disappearance of calcification in 15% of patients with radiologically proven calcification of the pancreas.

Zentler-Munro: Do gallstones in reality cause chronic pancreatitis or are they a consequence?

McMahon: The evidence that gallstones actually cause chronic pancreatitis is hard to find, in spite of the fact that it is confidently stated in many pre-1970 texts. There is no doubt that gallstone pancreatitis is much less acute than might be thought from the clinical presentation. At least 3 groups have demonstrated that there are abnormalities of pancreatic function lasting for as long as 6 months after an apparently short-lived attack of gallstone related pancreatitis.

IS THERE A ROLE FOR PANCREATIC FUNCTION TESTS IN THE EVALUATION OF CHRONIC PANCREATITIS?

Mr EJS Boyd
Senior Registrar
Glasgow Royal Infirmary

Introduction

Measurement of bicarbonate and enzyme concentrations in duodenal aspirate after stimlation of pancreatic exocrine secretion by exogenous secretagogues has been used for over 40 years in the evaluation of patients suspected to suffer from chronic pancreatitis. Indeed, a persistently abnormal secetory response to direct stimulation with exogenous secretagogues was previously considered a necessary diagnostic criterion for chronic pancreatitis. The development of improved pancreatic imaging techniques (endoscopic retrograde pancreatography (ERP), ultrasonography (US), and computerised tomography (CT) and tests of pancreatic exocrine function which do not require duodenal intubation, has meant that the role of direct pancreatic function testing in chronic pancreatitis has changed.

Pancreatic exocrine function may be measured in order to establish the presence of chronic pancreatic disease, by demonstrating impaired exocrine function, to establish the cause of the pancreatic hypofunction, to determine disease progression as an aid to prognosis, or to guide therapy.

ESTABLISHING DIAGNOSIS

The Secretin (+Cholecystokinin) Test. False positive results may occur in patients recovering from acute pancreatitis, after ERP, in severe coeliac disease, in diabetes mellitus, and after truncal vagotomy. If these conditions are excluded the specificity of an abnormal test is high - from 85-95%. The test may require to be repeated in order to confirm that the secretory impairment is persistent. The secretin (+CCK) test is less satisfactory for excluding chronic pancreatitis. The sensitivity has varied from 17% to 95% in reported series.

The Lundh Test. The Lundh test measures enzyme concentrations (rather than outputs) in the duodenal aspirate. The pH of the aspirate is only a crude indication of bicarbonate secretion by the pancreas. In comparison with the secretin (+CCK) test the Lundh test is less sensitive and specific. The lower specificity is attributable to a higher proportion of abnormal results occuring in patients with diabetes, coeliac disease, or obstructive jaundice, and in patients who have undergone previous gastric surgery.

The bentiromide and Pancreolauryl tests are approximatley equally sensitive and specific. When exocrine insufficency is sufficently severe to result in steatorrhoea the sensitivity of each test is 95-100%. However, in less severe exocrine insufficiency the sensitivity falls to 40 - 50%, a value which is insufficiently high for diagnostic purposes.

Serum trypsin and pancreatic isoamylase concentrations are related to the functional pancreatic acinar cell mass. However, it is only in advanced pancreatic exocrine insufficiency, accompanied by steatorrhoea and diabetes mellitus, that diagnostic sensitivities of over 90% occur.

Establishing the Cause of the Pancreatic Hypofunction

Both chronic pancreatitis and pancreatic cancer result in impaired exocrine pancreatic secretion. There is no characteristic pattern of secretory impairment in response to stimulation with secretin (+CCK) which permits differentiation between the two diseases. Similarly the Lundh test, oral function tests and serum enzyme concentrations cannot differentiate between pancreatic cancer and chronic pancreatitis as the cause of exocrine secretory impairment.

Carcinoembryonic antigen (CAE)

Pancreatic oncofoetal antigen (POA)

∝–Foeto protein (∝-FP)

Carbohydrate antigen 19-9 (CA19-9)

Carbohydrate antigen 50 (CA-50)

Tissue polypeptide antigen (TPA)

Table 1 Serum and pancreatic juice antigens used in the differentiation of chronic pancreatitis from pancreatic cancer

It is possible to obtain material for cytological examination from the duodenal aspirate during the secretin (+CCK) test in 39% to 87% of patients. Diagnostic sensitivity and specificity for pancreatic cancer have ranged from 14% to 60% and from 90% to 100% respectively. Estimation of lactoferrin concentrations in the duodenal aspirate or in pure pancreatic juice obtained at ERP is no longer considered to be helpful in differentiating pancreatitis from pancreatic cancer. A range of tumour antigens has been measured in duodenal aspirate or in the serum in an attempt to detect pancreatic cancer (Table 1). Serum concentrations are more discriminating and may allow advanced cancer to be differentiated from chronic pancreatitis. Tumour antigens do not appear to be of value in the detection of small (<3cms diameter) cancers.

DETERMINATION OF DISEASE PROGRESSION

Sequential secretin (+CCK) tests can provide evidence for disease progression, and have also been used to document improvement in pancreatic function with time following partial pancreatic resection, and in patients with alcoholic chronic pancreatitis who have stopped drinking. However, it appears that in patients with established chronic pancreatitis, non-invasive tests of exocrine function are reproducible and can be used more conveniently to document disease progress.

A GUIDE TO THERAPY

A reduction in pancreatic lipase output in response to CCK to less than 10% of normal has been reported to result in steatorrhoea, and to be an indication for treatment with pancreatic enzyme replacement therapy. However, enzyme output is only one determinant of fat digestion in pancreatic disease and maldigestion of fat may occur with near normal lipase secretion when there is gastric acid hypersecretion, rapid gastric emptying or interference with bile acid secretion. Conversely, some patients (particularly those in South Africa) appear to have normal fat digestion despite severely reduced lipase secretion. The Lundh test has been employed to determine the effects of gastric anti-secretory drugs and pancreatic enzyme supplementation on the concentrations of enzymes in the duodenal lumen. An improvement in PABA excretion following a variant of the bentiromide test has been used to determine the optimal dose of pancreatic enzyme supplements in children with cyctic fibrosis. Similarly the 13C- or 14C-triolein breath test may be used to document improvement in fat absorption during treatment with pancreatic enzyme supplements. In the majority of patients, however, clinical features such as weight gain and reduction in stool frequency are sufficient indices on which to base enzyme replacement therapy.

WHEN SHOULD PANCREATIC FUNCTION TESTS BE USED?

The diagnostic specificity and sensitivity of direct pancreatic function tests are similar to those of ERP and CT. However, ERP and CT are preferable initial investigations because only they can identify complications such as bile duct stenosis or pancreatic cysts, can provide unequivocal evidence for pancreatic cancer, and can be used to plan surgical procedures on the pancreas. If these imaging techniques are normal or equivocal, patients supected of suffering from chronic pancreatitis should undergo a secretin (+CCK) test, since in a small proportion of patients (about 9%) abnormalities of exocrine function may provide the only evidence for chronic pancreatitis. In a further7% of patients the diagnosis of chronic pancreatitis may only be made by biopsy at laparotomy or lesser-sac laparoscopy.

Mild ductal changes on ERP ("minimal change pancreatitis", "mild chronic pancreatitis") do not always indicate histological chronic pancreatitis. When histological examination has been undertaken in patients with minimal ERP changes only about half have had histological evidence of chronic pancreatitis. Patients with minimal ERP abnormalities should undergo further evaluation by the secetin (+CCK) test. Duodenal drainage studies are abnormal in about 50% of patients with mild ERP abnormalities and may thus provide confirmatory evidence for chronic pancreatitis.

Tubeless tests of pancreatic function are too insensitive to be of value in the diagnosis of chronic pancreatitis. However, they may be useful for documenting changes in exocrine function with time in patients with established chronic pancreatitis, and for assessing the effects of enzyme replacement therapy.

References:

1. EJS Boyd and KG Wormsley. Laboratory tests in the diagnosis of the chronic pancreatic diseases, Part 1: Secretagogues used in tests of pancreatic secretion, *Int J Pancreatol* 1987;2:137-148
2. EJS Boyd and KG Wormsley. Laboratory tests in the diagnosis of the chronic pancreatic diseases, Part 2: Tests of pancreatic secretion, *Int J Pancreatol* 1987;2:211-221
3. H Rinderknecht, EJS Boyd and KG Wormsley. Laboratory tests in the diagnosis of the chronic pancreatic diseases, Part 3: Tubeless test of pancreatic function, *Int J Pancreatol* 1987;2;281-293
4. EJS Boyd, H Rinderknecht and KG Wormsley. Laboratory tests in the diagnosis of the chronic pancreatic diseases, Part 4: Tests involving the measurement of pancreatic enzymes in body fluid, *Int J Pancreatol* 1988; 3:1-16
5. EJS Boyd and KG Wormsley. Laboratory tests in the diagnosis of the chronic pancreatic diseases, Part 5: Stool enzyme measurements, *Int J Pancreatol* 1988;3:101-103
6. EJS Boyd, H Rinderknecht and KG Wormsley. Laboratory tests in the diagnosis of the chronic pancreatic diseases, Part 6: Differentiation between chronic pancreatitis and pancreatic cancer, *Int J Pancreatol* 1988;3:229-240
7. EJS Boyd, H Rinderknecht and KG Wormsley. Laboratory tests in the diagnosis of the chronic pancreatic diseases, Part 7: Comparison between function tests and morphologic investigation in the diagnosis of pancreatic disease, *Int J Pancreatol* 1988;3:301-308

DISCUSSION

Imrie: How do you perform a direct test if secretin is unavailable?

Boyd: There is no product licence for secretin and CCK in Britain. The drugs can be acquired on a named patient basis: secretin from Hoechst in Frankfurt; synthetic secretin from Roche in Switzerland, and Serolin from Pharmitalia. It is a nuisance and can delay the test by 2 or 3 weeks.

Zentler-Munro: If you were setting up a new test, what would be your gold standard?

Boyd: In Dundee, the gold standard has been direct visualisation of the pancreas and histology. Histology has been the method in good secretin studies, for example, in the Way study, all the patients were operated on and had histology. In the Valentini study for probably 70-80% of those patients, histology was the final diagnostic arbiter.

Salmon: Histology is possible by fine needle aspiration. Dr Lees (Middlesex) has a large experience now, with perhaps 200 patients. It is safe, and can allow one to take biopsies from different parts of the pancreas.

McMahon: I am intrigued by the test advocated by Heptner et al, looking at amino acid consumption from the plasma in response to CCK and secretin.

Boyd: It is an interesting idea but has never been the subject of proper scientific analysis for its sensitivity. NMR scanning may prove useful, producing morphological and functional information on the same scan.

Russell : The initial results with that have not been very good, but I think a lot more work needs to be done. One needs a second or third generation NMR scanner to be able to achieve this level of differentiation.

Reference

1. Heptner G, Domschke S, Schneider MU, Kolb S, Domschke W. Amino acid level in plasma-expressed as alpha-amino-nitrogen - reaction to stimulation of the exocrine pancreas: approaches to a new pancreatic function test. Klin Wochenschr 1987; 65:1054-61.

THE FUTURE FOR SURGERY IN CHRONIC PANCREATITIS

Mr R C G Russell
Consultant Surgeon
The Middlesex Hospital
London

Introduction

The surgery of pancreatitis lacks definitions. There are no gold standards on which to base therapy, indications for operating or results of that surgical treatment. There is no evidence that medical management will change the course of the disease, unless more is learnt about the aetiology and pathogenesis of chronic pancreatitis.

For the moment surgery remains the main therapy for severe chronic pancreatitis. The surgeon must satisfy himself of the indications for surgery. In my own series, pain was the primary reason for intervention, being present in 99% of patients. Additionally, narcotic abuse leading to weight loss, loss of work, and the complications of the disease were frequently major indications for surgical treatment. The question is at what level of pain or narcotic abuse is operation indicated? Is intervention indicated before severe narcotic abuse occurs?

Anatomy and Aetiology

With the use of ERCP, ultrasound, and CT scanning, the state of the pancreas can be well imaged before operating. Minimal change pancreatitis has been discussed. Some of these patients do have extremely severe symptoms and doubt must be expressed as to whether they have pancreatitis or another disease, and whether the changes seen are the cause of pain. An annular pancreas and other congenital anomalies can give rise to pain on occasion. The Marseilles classification includes patients with obstructive pancreatitis, where there is an obstruction within the pancreatic duct, for example with calcific pancreatitis, and these patients can be treated adequately by surgery. Some patients present solely with duct dilatation frequently secondary to obstruction near the head of the pancreas.The clinical picture produced by such a complication of chronic pancreatitis may vary, but some sort of operative intervention will be indicated.

The aetiology can affect the indication for surgery. In our series of over 200 patients with chronic pancreatitis, 15 - 20% were caused directly by gallstones. The stones disrupt the pancreatic duct and produce pain, frequently of great severity. If the gall bladder is removed early these patients do not get further problems. There are therefore times when the threshold for operative intervention is lower. Patients with alcoholic pancreatitis, who continue to drink after surgical treatment of chronic pancreatitis tend to do badly. Hyperlipidemia, hypercalcemia and other rarer aetiologies can be corrected medically. The abnormalities in the duct may continue to cause symptoms, in which case the threshold for an operation will be less. Congenital anomalies, benign tumours, cysts, and various other aetiologies, which are increasingly recognised, can be treated by an appropriate operation with good results.

The questions to be answered are "Would early intervention prevent the progression of the disease?" and "Would early intervention prevent the addiction to narcotics?" The continuing pain syndrome is a major problem. Despite every sort of medical management, some patients have had pain for 7 to 10 years, and will take large amounts of narcotics. Whatever you do to that group, they seem to continue getting pain after their operation. Will better timing of operative intervention save narcotic abuse, and prevent the progression of the disease with its long-term sequelae? Alternatively if operation is undertaken too early, what problems may develop? The consequences of a partial gastrectomy are well recognised and a pancreatic resection frequently includes this, with loss of the duodenum as well as the removal of much of the pancreas. Will this have long-term sequelae which shortens the life of the patient? Will intervention lead to too many total pancreatectomies, with a life of diabetes and exocrine insufficiency which can be difficult to manage?fear this has happened.

NON - SURGICAL TECHNIQUES

The role of interventional radiology must be considered, especially in the management of complications such as abscess formation. Many pseudocysts can now be treated without recourse to surgery. Biopsy can be important where it is difficult to differentiate between benign and maligant conditions. Recently several fistulae have been cured by the use of somatostatin. Stones can be removed endoscopically with complete relief of the symptoms. Sphincterotomy of the pancreatic duct has been used, but apart from removing stones there have been no good long-term effects.

SURGICAL TECHNIQUES

Plugging of the pancreatic duct with various forms of glue has been attempted in order to induce a complete obliteration of the duct and atrophy of the acinar glands. This is still used in Germany, but my experience is not good.

An inappropriate procedure is one of the commonest causes for a poor surgical result. In retrospect many total pancreatectomies have resulted from performing a distal pancreatectomy where it would have been more appropriate to do a proximal pancreatectomy, and vice versa. Large series from German centres are quoting mortalities for pancreato-duodenectomy in the region of 1% to 1.5%. This must be the figure to aim for when dealing with benign disease in young people. The median age of our patients is 42 years. The future of surgery will depend on keeping the mortality rate low and reducing the morbidity to adequate levels.

The choice of surgical procedures is worthy of mention: drainage procedures come first and sphincteroplasty has a time honoured place. For the major duct the latter has no place, but in pancreas divisum an accessory sphincterotomy is probably the first procedure that should be done, and I find 50% of patients benefit. Duct drainage remains the ideal procedure as it prevents the reduction of acinar tissue, and more importantly, islet tissue. It is only of value if the duct diameter is greater than one centimetre. The surgical technique is important because the duct has to be opened from the head of the pancreas to the tail, in other words, about 10-15 centimetres. Many suggest that it should be possible to pass probes from the head of the pancreas into the duodenum without difficulty to ensure that you have relieved all the obstructive elements in that area. Distal resection has had a bad name, but it is the ideal procedure if the disease is confined to the body and tail of the pancreas. This is often the case where the complications of acute pancreatitis have given rise to a chronic disease process, or in those groups with recurrent acute pancreatitis due to obstruction or partial obstruction in the body of the pancreas. The long-term results with distal resection are far better than with proximal resection. Longmire advocated that chronic pancreatitis arises in the head of the pancreas due to a disruption of the ductal drainage system. Accordingly many patients with the more severe disease undergo a resection at the head of the pancreas. A decision regarding the appropriate resection can only be made by carefully documenting the patients, and by examining them with all modalities of imaging to determine where the major disease lies. Total pancreatectomy should be reserved for a very small group of patients who have severe problems following previous treatment. It should not be the primary surgical procedure.

Conclusion

The surgical management of chronic pancreatitis will only advance when the disease is better understood. It is important to select patients more carefully, to fit the operation to the particular disease with which one is dealing, and to realise that long-term care is very important. The endocrine and exocrine deficiency that many of these patients will develop will mean that follow-up has to continue for the lifetime of the patient.

DISCUSSION

Trapnell: Is there any force in Rudi Ammann's argument that this disease can burn itself out? Is this a geographic variation or a facet of a different aetiology to account for his observation? Alcoholic pancreatitis in the UK and America is, for instance, very different.

Imrie: I do not think so. Even in Ammann's studies quite a number of patients receive surgery for pain control, but his papers focus on the group who do not. Having a reputation of advising patients that their pain will spontaneously resolve within 8 or 10 years must certainly affect one's referrals.

Russell: I agree, we have followed a large number of people in our clinic for as long as ten years. The pattern of their disease does not change over that time, nor have I found a patient in which the disease has burnt itself out without any intervention. Even those who genuinely stop alcohol and get relief from pain initially, develop symptoms again, later.

Jones: In the relatively sober Weald of Kent we find little chronic pancreatitis. Are we missing it and is it very variable in the way it presents?

Russell: The presentation is very consistent. There is marked regional variation, the alcohol consumption in the south of England is not small, and yet we do not see a large amount of alcohol related chronic pancreatitis. I do not understand this. Many of our patients have other aetiologies and one must stress the care needed to investigate the person in order to find the underlying cause.

Taylor: You said that continuing to drink alcohol was a contraindication to surgery? Why is that the case if it does not make any difference to prognosis.

Russell: To help future management: diabetic alcoholics can be very difficult to control.

Taylor: When the gland is confluently involved with disease of similar severity in the head, body and tail, and when there is not gross dilatation of the duct to a centimetre or more, how do you choose between a distal pancreatectomy, a total pancreatectomy or a resection of the head?

Russell: These patients with diffuse disease appear to do badly with a distal pancreatectomy. I would preserve the body and tail and see if they settle.

Taylor: Is the mechanism of pain understood in chronic pancreatitis?

Imrie: No, and the fact that a number of patients who have had total pancreatectomies continue with a similar pain is disturbing.

Russell: We have a number of patients with continued pain following pancreatectomy. We have found that with care and careful reduction of their narcotic therapy the pain resolves.

McMahon: I have been impressed how malignant the disease can be in women. Have you noticed a relationship with gender?

Russell: Yes, we have a curious female group who have minimal change pancreatitis with a fibrosed, thickened gland, which causes immense pain which we have really been unsuccessful in managing. This group will continue getting pain even after a total pancreatectomy.

Taylor: Do you use nerve blockade before pancreatectomy or following unsatisfactory results?

Russell: We have largely given up nerve blockade. It is immensely useful in those with cancer of the pancreas, but with chronic pancreatitis, the effect rapidly wears off; three to four months benefit from the first administration, one to two from the next, and thereafter it becomes totally ineffective.

Boyd: Is the objection to these patients becoming narcotic addicts entirely a moral or religous one?

Russell: No. We have several people in that category consuming up to 2 grams of pethidine daily. Several problems develop. At these very high doses, some patients have developed epileptiform fits, which at present remain unexplained. Additionally four patients developed a form of Wernicke's encephalopathy which was thought initially to be due to thiamine deficiency secondary to their suspected alcoholism. Surprisingly thiamine supplements made no difference, they were shown not to be alcoholics, and they recovered spontaneously after six to nine months. These two groups appear to differ as the former did not develop the long tract signs of the latter. The causes for both however remain a mystery.

Imrie: Mr Russell, duct plugging is now carried out only in Erlangen, where they appear to perform one Whipple's operation a week. Do you not think it is very difficult to equate their results with most other centres? If one operates on all patients showing the slightest suggestion of chronic pancreatitis, then one should have a low mortality.

Boyd: Certainly there is a great keeness to operate in Germany. This is well shown by the larger overall number of duodenal-preserving operations performed.

Jones: Mr Russell, you were suggesting the fillet type of procedure in those patients with dilatation of the duct greater than one centimetre. Lord Smith advocates the alternative procedure of a more straight forward pancreatico- jejunostomy without doing the fillet procedure. Is there good evidence now to suggest that the longer anastomosis that you describe is superior?

Russell : Bradley in the United States has looked at this in detail. If the pancreatico- jejunostomy is less than 6 centimetres, they work poorly, greater than 6 centimetres the results are good. My experience with any form of pancreatico- jejunostomy is that the anastomosis blocks and I have the greatest difficulty in keeping them patent. I would suspect the majority of those that Lord Smith performed did block off, although this may take as long as one to three years.

PAIN RELIEF IN CHRONIC PANCREATITIS - A PHYSIOLOGICAL APPROACH

Dr P L Zentler-Munro
Consultant Physician
Raigmore Hospital
Inverness

The relief of pain in chronic pancreatitis is notoriously difficult to achieve. Many patients suffer severe pain despite taking large doses of opiate analgesics, and some suffer associated problems of habituation. Neurolytic procedures seldom achieve lasting relief of pain, whilst pancreatic resection extensive enough to assuredly relieve pain can produce a diabetic state with which many patients particularly those habituated to alcohol or analgesics - cannot cope.

For many years, however, some physicians have toyed with the use of pancreatic enzyme supplementation as treatment for chronic pancreatic pain - a form of drug therapy which, whether or not effective, is at least entirely safe, inexpensive and "natural". The rationale for this treatment is based on a physiological model of the control of pancreatic secretion which was at first no more than a rational assumption, but over the years has graduated into a hypothesis and, in some parts, to empirical observation. This model has not been applied quantitavely to suggest exactly how such treatment should be given, and recent advances suggesting how it might be optimised have not been exploited. The treatment itself is used in few centres and has not been subjected to adequate clinical trial.

I propose here, therefore, to present a model of one aspect of the control of pancreatic exocrine secretion, and to discuss how its practical application to treatment could best be validated.

PHYSIOLOGICAL CONTROL OF PANCREATIC ENDOCRINE SECRETION

It seems sensible to suppose that the presence of pancreatic enzymes in the duodenum above a certain concentration inhibits the secretion of further enzymes from the pancreas. This has been demonstrated in many animals, as has the converse - that a reduction in intraduodenal enzyme activity stimulates pancreatic secretion. Animal studies are of limited relevance to man, due to important species differences, and are not discussed further here.

Evidence for such a negative feedback in normal man is more controversial. Diversion of pancreato-biliary fluid away from the duodenum and subsequent reinfusion stimulates and inhibits respectively pancreatic secretion. (1) Of the many factors in pancreato-biliary fluid which could immediate this, pancreatic protease has the best credentials. Studies in healthy man have shown that infusion of trypsin into the duodenum inhibits the secretion of pancreatic enzymes (2) in response to ingestion of a mixed meal, or infusion of phenylalanine or oleic acid (3) but not in response to a volume (saline) or osmotic stimulus. (4) Infusion of lipase or amylase has no such effect. (3) The inhibition may be initiated only in the duodenum, since infusion of pancreatic juice into the jejunum does not inhibit saline- stimulated pancreatic secretion ,(5) although this may by an inappropriate stimulus. Administration of a trypsin inhibitor, conversely, stimulated pancreatic enzyme secretion in some (2,6) but not all (7,8) studies. The absence of an effect in the latter studies could have been due to the use of aprotinin as an inhibitor - which has little effect on chymotrypsin - or to the use of a weak stimulus to pancreatic enzyme secretion; inhibition of basal intraduodenal trypsin may not stimulate the feedback mechanism. The most recent and convincing positive study (6) used an inhibitor of both enzymes and collected pure pancreatic juice.

It might also seem reasonable to suppose that the presence of bile acid in the duodenum might suppress further gall bladder contraction and hence pancreatic acinar secretion, since the secretagogue is shared - cholecystokinin (CCK). This negative feedback mechanism has been demonstrated in a perfusion experiment using taurocholate at physiological concentrations (9) and also, more recently, using oral UDCA .(10) These studies point to a convenient, safe and equally "natural" way of amplifying the effect of protease, by administration of UDCA as widely used in gallstone dissolution therapy.

The negative feedback is, in both cases, most probably mediated in part by CCK - a hormone that is secreted predominantly from duodenal mucosa. Although one would not expect necessarily to detect any effect in systemic venous blood, studies have shown that intraduodenal infusion of trypsin (3,4) but not lipase or amylase (3) reduces stimulated CCK levels. The converse effect - an increase in CCK after pancreatobiliary diversion or the use of a trypsin inhibitor has been demonstrated in animals but not in man .(11)

A second and separate negative feedback probably exists in healthy man, and operates via a cholinergic mechanism in response to different stimuli. Stimulation of pancreatic enzyme secretion with a duodenal volume or osmotic load is unaccompanied by any rise in CCK, and is inhibited by intravenous atropine but not by intraduodenal trypsin. (4) The CCK response to phenylalanine is, conversely, inhibited by trypsin but not by atropine; the pancreatic secretory response is blocked to the greatest extent by both together (4) suggesting that both mechanisms may operate together in physiological responses. The use of an oral anticholinergic drug in the treatment of chronic pancreatitis is less attractive, even though one such drug - pirenzepine - is claimed to be specific for muscarinic receptors in the upper gut.

PATHOPHYSIOLOGICAL CONTROL OF PANCREATIC EXOCRINE SECRETION

Application of this model to chronic pancreatitis would suggest that a reduction in the secretion of pancreatic enzymes and concomitant reduction in their intraduodenal concentration would stimulate CCK release and thus acinar secretion. This secretion would occur into damaged pancreatic ductules with reduced compliance and increased resistance to flow, leading to increased intraductular pressure and reflux of potent hydrolytic enzymes into pancreatic acini and resultant cell damage. Although little is known of the pathogenesis of pain in chronic pancreatitis, there is some evidence that ductular hypertension may contribute, whilst acinar damage might well do particularly if local inflammatory mediator were released. The resultant acinar damage would further impair pancreatic enzyme secretion, resulting in a vicious circle which would be interrupted only when the patient developed end-stage pancreatic fibrosis and associated achylia.

Evidence for this model is sparse but increasing. The negative feedback loop appears to be intact, since, as in health, intraduodenal infusion of trypsin 10g/l (but not lipase or amylase) reduced amino acid-induced pancreatic secretion in patients with relatively preserved pancreatic function, and co-administration of a trypsin inhibitor reversed this inhibition. (12) These effects were not seen in patients with chronic pancreatitis sufficiently severe to cause steatorrhoea. The effect of bile acid in chronic pancreatitis has not been studied.

Whether the feedback actually operates physiologically is less clear. Although reduced secretion of pancreatic enzymes into the duodenum is the diagnostic hallmark of chronic pancreatitis, intraduodenal concentrations of trypsin are not always decreased - as reflected in the relative insensitivity of the Lundh test to mild disease. Plasma CCK levels in patients with chronic pancreatitis are highly controversial, due in part to methodological problems with the early bile assay of this hormone, and more recently problems with gastrin crossreactivity in the immunoassay. Three recent studies have identified increased CCK levels, one using an antibody suspected of crossreaction (13) and the others using a more specific antibody .(14,15) The increases appeared greater in those with relatively preserved exocrine function. Two equally careful studies, however, one using the same antibody (16) and the other using antibodies to three different areas of the CCK molecule (17) found no evidence of increase, but the patients mostly had advanced pancreatic insufficiency. The study using the less specific antibody to identify an increase, also showed that administration of pancreatin reduced the elevated levels .(13)

It should be noted, however, that this model does not require that the negative feedback be intensified in chronic pancreatitis, but simply that it operate in the presence of decreased ductular compliance or flow. Systemic blood levels of CCK may be irrelevant to the feedback system, since CCK may diffuse directly from duodenum to pancreas.

More importantly, these studies have failed to give any clear indication of what oral dose of trypsin is needed to achieve maximal suppression of enzyme secretion. Perfusion experiments in healthy man have shown maximal (40%) suppression of amino acid- stimulated secretion at a trypsin concentration of 1.0g/l (4) but in chronic pancreatitis a higher concentration (2.5g/1) is needed (12). These levels are higher than those of endogenous trypsin present in normal postprandial duodenal aspirate, suggesting a pharmacological rather than purely physiological response. It appears that both trypsin and chymotrypsin may be needed, since inhibition of trypsin alone in health - where both enzymes are secreted - has no effect. (7,8) The enzymes may also have to be present in enzymatically active form, since inhibition of the catalytic site of trypsin suppressed its inhibitory effect. (12) Both these observations suggest that the final mediator might be a digestive product (common to both proteases), but this seems unlikely as no obvious substrate was included in most of the studies. There has been no study of the effect of bile acid therapy or of pirenzepine on pancreatic secretion in chronic pancreatitis.

CLINICAL TRIALS

Despite the empirical doubts about the validity of the model, rational conviction seems to have led many physicians to try the treatment in clinical practice, and a few to test it in clinical trials. Pancreatin, in various formulations, has been used as a source of trypsin; its use to treat steatorrhoea in chronic pancreatitis (18) is well established, and its use to treat pain, in patients without steatorrhoea, therefore all the more convenient.

Four randomised placebo-controlled clinical trials have been reported, none of them adequate in design and none large enough to have a high probability of detecting a worthwhile reduction in pain - the largest included only 20 patients. Despite the differing designs, durations, treatments and assessments used in these trials, certain messages emerge. In both the positive trials (12,19) women and those with idiopathic pancreatitis tended to respond better and, in the one which considered the problem, (12) those with a better preserved pancreatic function and without steatorrhoea responded better. Reduction in pain score was impressive - by about 70% in at least 50% of patients in both trials - but only the longer trial allowing one month per treatment (12) demonstrated a reduction in analgesic requirements. One of the two negative trials allowed only two weeks per treatment and used a very low dose of pancreatin (2 capsules per meal), although sufficient to reduce fat excretion in those with steatorrhoea. (20) The other (21) appeared to select only patients who had previously not responded to pancreatin. No trial has assessed the efficacy of bile acid therapy or of an anticholinergic drug, with or without pancreatin, in this area. All of the trials illustrate the difficulty of defining pancreatic pain in chronic pancreatitis, and of distinguishing it from pain due to malabsorption and ensuing bowel dysmotility. Some have argued that if pancreatin has any effect on pain, it is on the latter rather than the former form. It is clear, however, that the response in those without underlying steatorrhoea (12) and the absence of change in bowel habit (19) or in colonic transit (20) refute this criticism.

Certain other problems emerge. Two of the trials determined the dose in relation to the concentrations in duodenal perfusate needed to suppress secretion (12) or to achieve improved intraduodenal levels (19) but no attempts to demonstrate its adequacy in each individual by showing suppression of CCK levels. Nor is it known whether the trypsin survives passage through the stomach (if uncoated) to be released early enough in the duodenum (if enteric coated) (18) in active form. All trials use a randomised placebo controlled crossover design but the limbs may not be long enough for achievement of steady state either in pancreatic secretion or in analgesic consumption. The latter is particularly important, as analgesic consumption offers a convenient and relevant means of assessing treatment efficacy in addition to pain scores. Many patients, however, are habituated to potent analgesics and it may take several weeks for them to reduce their consumption in response to a successful treatment. If the first treatment is effective in reducing analgesic consumption, it would then be necessary to provide a washout period between treatments to allow analgesic consumption to rise to its untreated level prior to testing the companion treatment.

Blinding is clearly essential, but difficult to achieve given the distinctive taste of pancreatin even in microsphere formulations. One trial (19) circumvented this problem by using heat- inactivated pancreatin as placebo. Reduction of steatorrhoea, if present, will unmask any placebo and for this and other reasons already discussed, it may be better to exclude patients with steatorrhoea from clinical trials.

It is clearly important that such "antisecretory" treatment be tested in clinical trials rather than offered on the basis of a theoretical model, since an opposite model can also be advanced: that pain in chronic pancreatitis is in part due to maldigestion and could be treated by stimulating rather than inhibiting pancreatic secretion. There is no pathophysiological study to support this model, but two trials studying the effect of prolonged treatment with intranasal CCK-octapeptide (22) and with a trypsin inhibitor (23) in patients with chronic pancreatitis noted a prolonged improvement in pancreatic secretory function and in symptoms. Unfortunately, the nature of the symptoms is not described in either report, and it is not clear whether true pancreatic pain, or more minor non-specific or maldigestive symptoms, was ameliorated.

Conclusion

What little is known of the pathophysiology of pain in chronic pancreatitis suggests that inhibition of the pancreatic acinar secretion may reduce pancreatic pain. The presence of either pancreatic protease or bile acid in the duodenum inhibits cholecystokinin release and reduces pancreatic acinar secretion in health. This pharmacological negative feedback can be demonstrated in patients with chronic pancreatitis, but whether it operates physiologically is not yet clear. Its existence does, however, point to a simple, safe, natural and inexpensive form of therapy for chronic pancreatic pain - pancreatin with or without bile acid.

Despite the obvious attraction of this form of therapy, it has not been tested adequately in clinical trials or, probably, exploited effectively in clinical practice. It is time that this deficiency was corrected.

References

1 . Boyd E J S, Cumming J G R, Cushieri A, Wormsley K G. Aspects of feedback control of pancreatic secretion in man. *Ital J Gastroenterol* 1985; 17: 18-22.
2. Ihse I, Lilja P, Lundquist I. Feedback regulation of pancreatic enzyme secretion by intestinal trypsin in man. *Digestion* 1977; 15: 303-8.
3. Owyang C, Louie D S, Tatum D. Feeback regulation of pancreatic enzyme secretion - suppression of cholecystokinin release by trypsin. *J Clin Invest* 1986; 77: 2042-7.
4. Owyang C, May D,Louie D S. Trypsin suppression of pancreatic enzyme secretion - differential effect on cholecystokinin release and the enteropancreatic reflex. *Gastroenterology* 1986; 91 : 637- 43.
5. Krawisz B R, Miller L J, DiMagno E P, Go V L W. In the absence of nutrients, pancreatic-biliary secretions in the jejunum do not exert feedback control of human pancreatic or gastric function. *J Lab Clin Med* 1980; 95: 13-18.
6. Liener I E, Goodale R L, Deshmukh A et al. Effect of a trypsin inhibitor from soybeans (Bowman-Birk) on the secretory activity of the human pancreas. *Gastroenterology* 1988; 94: 419-27.
7. Hotz J, Ho S B, Go V L W, DiMagno E P. Short-term inhibition of duodenal tryptic activity does not affect human pancreatic, biliary or gastric function. J Lab Clin Med 1983; 101 : 488-95.
8. Dlugosz J, Folsch U R, Creutzfeldt W. Inhibition of intraduodenal trypsin does not stimulate exocrine pancreatic secretion in man. *Digestion* 1983; 26: 197-204.
9. Malagelada J R, Go V L W, DiMagno E P, Summerskill W H J.Interactions between intraluminal bile acids and digestive products on pancreatic and gallbladder function. *J Clin Invest* 1973; 52: 2160-5.
10. Lanzini A, Hall N, Facchinetti D, Northfield T C. Effect of ursodeoxycholic acid (UDCA) on pancreatin enzyme secretion and gall bladder emptying. *Clin Sci* 1987; 72: 31-31 (abstract).
11 . Folsch U R, Wilms H, Schafmayer A, Becker H D, Creutzfeldt W. The negative feedback mechanism of pancreatic enzyme secretion is accompanied by elevated CCK plasma concentrations. *Dig Dis Sci* 1984; 29: 949 (abstract).
12. Slaff J, Jacobson D, Tillman C R, Curington C, Toskes P. Protease-specific suppression of pancreatic exocrine secretion. *Gastroenterology* 1984; 87: 44-52.
13. Slaff J I, Wolfe M, Toskes P P. Elevated fasting cholecytokinin levels in pancreatic exocrine impairment: Evidence to support feedback regulation. *J Lab Clin Med* 1985; 105: 282-5.
14. Funakoshi A, Nakano I, Shinozaki H, Tateishi K, Hamaoka T, Ibayashi H. High plasma cholecystokinin levels in patients with chronic pancreatitis having abdominal pain. *Am J Gastroenterol* 1986; 81: 1174-8.

15. Schafmayer A, Becker H D, Werner M, Folsch U R, Creutzfeldt W. Plasma cholecytokinin levels in patients with chronic pancreatitis. *Digestion* 1985 32: 136-9.
16. Cantor P, Petronijevic L, Worning H. Plasma cholecystokinin in patients with advanced chronic pancreatitis. *Pancreas* 1986; 1 : 488-93 .
17. Jansen J B M J, Hopman W P M, Lamers C B H W. Plasma cholecystkinin concentrations in patients with pancreatic insufficiency measured by sequence-specific radioimmunoassays. *Dig Dis Sci* 1984; 29: 1101-17.
18. Zentler-Munro P L, Northfield T C. Pancreatic enzyme replacement applied physiology and pharmacology. Aliment Pharmacol Therap 1987; 1: 575-92.
19. Isaksson G, Ihse I. Pain reduction by an oral pancreatic enzyme preparation in chronic pancreatitis. *Dig Dis Sci* 1983; 28: 97-102.
20. Halgreen H, Pedersen N T, Worning H. Symptomatic effect of pancreatic enzyme therapy in patients with chronic pancreatitis. *Scand J Gastroenterol* 1986; 21 : 104-8.
21. Armbrecht U, Svanvik J, Stockbrugger R. Enzyme substitution in chronic pancreatitis: Effects on clinical and functional parameters and on the hydrogen (H2) breath test. *Scand J Gastroenterol* 1986; 21 (Suppl 126): 55-9.
22. Pap A, Berger Z, Varro V. Trophic effect of cholecystokinin in man - a new way in the treatment of chronic pancreatitis? Digestion 1981; 21: 163-8. Pap A, Berger Z, Varro V. Benefician effect of a soy flour diet in chronic pancreatitis. *Mount Sinai J Med* 1983; 50: 208-12.
23. Pap A, Berger Z, Varro V. Benefician effect of a soy flour diet in chronic pancreatitis. Mount Sinai J Med 1983; 50: 208-12.

DISCUSSION

Boyd: Papp conducted two trials designed to increase CCK release in these patients and stimulate what was left of the pancreas. He found an improvement in exocrine function and symptoms. In the first he used raw soya flour for three days and in the second CCK octopeptide given intranasally. Does this not conflict with your hypothesis?

Zentler-Munro: The real question with the first study was, what was the soya bean doing? Food as a whole stimulates trypsin secretion and CCK release. Whether the soya bean trypsin inhibitor was actually doing anything in that experiment I do not know. I do not remember well the details of the pain side of the study, nor the effect of the intranasal CCK,but I think you will agree that the other studies that I have mentioned arouse interest.

Russell: In patients with steatorrhoea following a resection which involves the duodenum, up to 80 or 100 creon capsules a day may be required to free them of their diarrhoea. The dose varies enormously. One ought to be able to vary the dose to see which suits the patient.

Zentler-Munro: I have suggested the dose of enzyme because one is not trying to correct steatorrhoea, but simply achieve a normal level of trypsin in the duodenum. Having calculated the volume of acid and pancreatic secretion one can work out the dose of lipase required, which is in the region of 50,000 units, equivalent to 5 Creon capsules. If this is increased slightly to be on the safe side, the dose should be about 7 or 8 capsules of Creon. The control of steatorrhoea is another physiological event altogether where one is concerned not only with digestion but with solubilisation and mucosal absorption, and is much more complicated.

Another problem in correcting steatorrhoea is that there may be a rapid transit of a capsule whose coating takes time, 20 minutes or so, to dissolve at pH6 and whose pancreatin core then takes a further 30-40 minutes to disintegrate and release the enzymes into the environment. That is a long period of time in a shortened small bowel with a loss of the pylorus. I think many of these patients would do better with H2 blockade plus crude encapsulated powder, such as Pancrex V capsules.

Russell: We have used H2 blockade and powder rather than the coated preparation but there seems to be very little difference.

Imrie: Our experience with patients with chronic pancreatitis parallels Mr Russell's. The dose recommendations in the British National Formulary do not bear any resemblance to the real situation. It is too easy to blame the patient for a lack of compliance when in fact it is poor medicine and bad information that is the cause of the problem with the management of chronic pancreatitis. I do think these patients tend to be unreliable but it is compounded by the medical profession giving the wrong advice, especially to doctors unfamiliar with this group of patients.

If the patients find that the pancreatic supplements control or influence their pain they will regulate the dose. Furthermore, because they find it inconvenient to carry about pocketfuls of the preparation and upsetting to visit their local chemist and collect a trolley full of capsules, they will try to reduce the dose or even stop taking it if they can.

Russell: Our experience also is that they will vary their doses fairly sensibly. There is a trial running at present organised by Duphar which does show that these patients will keep their records, provided that you see them fortnightly and show interest in their diary cards. The major difficulty in managing a long study is that the disease is not static. I do not think it possible to choose a patient with a steady state of pain, which is why the Duphar trial has taken so long to accrue sufficient numbers.

Jones: Did you find a difference in the pancreatic supplement requirements between those patients who had had a pancreatectomy for chronic pancreatitis and those for other causes?

Russell: The overall variation in dose requirement has been from zero to 125 capsules per day. Even amongst the total pancreatectomies some patients need as little as 5 and some need around 100 capsules per day; it is very variable.

I am not sure why this extreme variability occurs. There are a lot of variables that one would like to measure, such as acid secretion and intraluminal pH. We have compared the results of different sorts of pancreatectomies but the numbers are small.

Imrie: The whole concept of chronic pancreatitis will change as people look at the disease more closely. Most doctors have been trained to see the patients with chronic pancreatitis in a way which bears little resemblance to the real person they meet. Many hold the view that these patients will weigh six and a half or seven and a half stone and be in constant pain. The truth is many are reasonably healthy looking people, and yet at ERCP there may be astonishing deformities of the gland which do cause pain.

Russell: To run this type of trial one needs well staffed pancreatic follow-up clinics. Patients distributed throughout general clinics are difficult to follow and treat. One needs a large population to cut down the number of centres. The patients wil respond well to doctors who are interested in them and will attend fortnightly. The support needed is very time consuming. We have an incredibly conscientious nurse who will spend about 4 hours a day on the telephone to our patients. This could not work for a national trial without some face to face contact.

PANCREATITIS ROUND TABLE
28th October 1988

DISCUSSANTS	AUDIENCE
Foster P N Leeds	Jones P A Kent
Hatfield A R W London	Kingsnorth A N Liverpool
Leese T Leicester	Larvin M Leeds
Shorvon P London	London N J M Leicester
	Northfield T C London
	Taylor T V Manchester